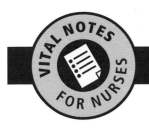

Professional Development, Reflection and Decision-making

Melanie Jasper

With contributions from Georgina Koubel, Gary Rolfe and Paul Elliott

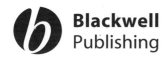

Blackwell
Publishing

© 2006 by Melanie Jasper

Blackwell Publishing editorial offices:
Blackwell Publishing Ltd, 9600 Garsington Road, Oxford OX4 2DQ, UK
    Tel: +44 (0)1865 776868
Blackwell Publishing Inc., 350 Main Street, Malden, MA 02148-5020, USA
    Tel: +1 781 388 8250
Blackwell Publishing Asia Pty Ltd, 550 Swanston Street, Carlton, Victoria
3053, Australia
    Tel: +61 (0)3 8359 1011

The right of the Author to be identified as the Author of this Work has been
asserted in accordance with the Copyright, Designs and Patents Act 1988.

First published 2006 by Blackwell Publishing Ltd

ISBN-13: 978-1-4051-3261-9
ISBN-10: 1-4051-3261-2

Library of Congress Cataloging-in-Publication Data
    Jasper, Melanie.
    Professional development, reflection, and decision-making / Melanie
Jasper ; with contributions from Georgina Koubel, Gary Rolfe, and Paul
Elliot.
        p. ; cm. – (Vital notes for nurses)
    Includes bibliographical references and index.
    ISBN-13: 978-1-4051-3261-9 (pbk. : alk. paper)
    ISBN-10: 1-4051-3261-2 (pbk. : alk. paper)
    1. Nursing.   2. Nursing–Decision making.   3. Reflection (Philosophy)
I. Title.   II. Series. [DNLM: 1. Nursing.   2. Decision Making.
3. Evidence-Based Medicine.   4. Nursing Theory. WY 16 J39p 2006]
    RT42.J37 2006
    610.73–dc22
    2006012265

A catalogue record for this title is available from the British Library

Set in 10/12 pt Palatino
by SNP Best-set Typesetter Ltd., Hong Kong
Printed and bound in Singapore
by Markono Print Media Pte Ltd

The publisher's policy is to use permanent paper from mills that operate a
sustainable forestry policy, and which has been manufactured from pulp
processed using acid-free and elementary chlorine-free practices.
Furthermore, the publisher ensures that the text paper and cover board used
have met acceptable environmental accreditation standards.

For further information on Blackwell Publishing, visit our website:
www.blackwellnursing.com

Contents

About the authors

Paul Elliott, MA, BSc, PGCEA, RGN, FRIPH, FRSH, MRCN, Assoc ICNA, MHEA
Senior Lecturer, Canterbury Christ Church University
The first half of my professional career was spent in the Royal Air Force undertaking a variety of duties culminating in an emergency nurse practitioner, aeromedical evacuation and battlefield nursing role with squadrons of front-line tactical support helicopters. In 1985 I left the Air Force and entered the National Health Service where I worked primarily within the accident and emergency and medical admissions settings. In 1991 I entered full-time health care education, this being the area in which my career has developed. I hold a Bachelor of Science degree in psychological studies and a Master's degree centring on the psychosocial aspects of infection control. My research interests lie within the psychosocial aspects of infection control and professional health care practice and I have a number of publications in these areas. I am a Fellow of the Royal Institute of Public Health and the Royal Society for the Promotion of Health.

Melanie Jasper, PhD, MSc, BNurs, BA, PGCEA, RGN, RM, RHV, NDN cert
Professor and Head of Health and Social Welfare Studies, Canterbury Christ Church University
Having practised in the community as a midwife and health visitor for a number of years post-qualification I moved into education as a senior lecturer at the University of Portsmouth in 1990. I was fortunate to be involved in many of the developments in nurse education throughout the next decade, including the recognition of nursing as a subject worthy of preparation at degree, Master's and doctoral levels, and the acknowledgement of nursing as a profession in its own right, necessi-

tating the development of critical, analytical and reflective skills for practice. During my time at Portsmouth I had the privilege of working closely with Gary Rolfe, now Professor of Nursing at University of Swansea. Together, we ventured into the realms of creating strategies to enable nurses to broaden their understanding of nursing practice by developing programmes that helped them to build on their previous experiences and to challenge and develop the knowledge base from which they practise.

Georgina Koubel, CQSW, KAPT, MSc Health and Community Studies
Senior Lecturer in Social Work, Canterbury Christ Church University
Having completed my certificate of qualification in social work in the mid-seventies, I took up the post of generic social worker in an inner London borough, working with a wide range of individuals and families. This involved working in areas of child protection, adoption and fostering and working with people with mental health difficulties and diverse disabilities. This led to a post in a hospital setting where I further developed my interests in counselling and collaborative working. I then worked for a while in voluntary agencies specialising in work with disadvantaged children, until I moved to Kent in 1993.

I became a care manager in the area of adult services (disabilities) with Kent County Council, where I developed a special interest in risk management and adult protection. While there, I qualified as a practice teacher and from there took a special interest in adult learning and student development. I also worked with colleagues at Canterbury Christ Church University to deliver a programme for nurse-trained care managers working within social services, which formed the basis for the adult services post-qualifying framework which I developed during my time as training manager (adult services) with KCC while undertaking my MSc in Health and Community Studies. As this neared completion, I took up the post of senior lecturer in the social work team on the inter-professional social work degree programme at Canterbury Christ Church University where I take the lead on adult services (discourses around older people and disability, which I also teach at Master's level), collaborative practice, social policy, community care law, care management, social work ethics and values and reflective practice.

Gary Rolfe, PhD, MA, BSc, RMN, PGCEA
Professor of Nursing, School of Health Science, University of Wales, Swansea
After qualifying as a mental health nurse in 1983, I worked for several years in acute psychiatric care and substance misuse, during which time I first became involved in clinical supervision and reflective prac-

tice. Following a short and exhausting spell as a lecturer practitioner, I moved into a full-time lecturing post at the University of Portsmouth, where I taught reflective practice and worked with Melanie Jasper on a number of innovative curriculum development projects. I currently teach and research in the field of practice development and have a particular interest in the challenges encountered by nurses in attempting to implement evidence-based practice.

The context of professional development

Learning objectives

This chapter explores the basis of professional development as an ongoing component of professional practice. It lays the foundations for the rest of the concepts in this book by exploring the context in which registered nurses, midwives and specialist community public health nurses work as accountable practitioners. It explores the responsibilities of nurses in terms of their own professional development, as lifelong learners and as practitioners belonging to a specific professional group. Finally, it presents a simple strategy for guiding professional development activities.

By the end of this chapter you will have:

- an understanding of the context within which professional development is framed
- considered your own professional development in relation to the Nursing and Midwifery Council's standards for continuing professional development
- an understanding of the nature of professional development from pre-registration to expert practice
- considered a range of professional development activities
- considered key mechanisms for professional development
- considered professional development within the context of lifelong learning
- used a strategy for identifying your professional development needs.

The context of professional development, reflective practice and decision-making

This book brings together the topics of professional development, reflective practice and decision-making. These concepts are all inextricably linked, as professional development is as much a cognitive process as it is a technical one. Reflective practice informs our decision-making as functioning professionals; learning to make decisions on the basis of our knowledge and experience results in evidence-based practice, and the identification of our knowledge and skills deficits, thus resulting in opportunities for development. Professional development means to advance ourselves as professional practitioners. It assumes that all professionals will continue to develop throughout their working lives – from becoming a student practitioner, to specialised and advanced practice. It assumes that they will progress beyond the levels of competence assumed at registration and qualification (Benner 1984) and become proficient, or even expert practitioners.

This development does not happen by accident, nor does it happen solely through formal educational processes, although these are certainly part of the way we continually acquire new knowledge and skills to inform our practice. The main ways in which we develop professionally, however, are through the practice of our profession itself, and the stimulation from the practice world that makes us continually build on our existing knowledge, seek out new knowledge and skills, make connections between our knowledge base and the challenges we encounter in practice, and learn from our experiences. Thus, professional practice and professional development are interdependent – our practice won't develop unless we develop as professionals. This is experiential learning, and will consciously arise from reflective practice – in turn it informs our decision-making. Hence, the links between professional development, reflective practice and decision-making can be represented as a triangle, seen in Figure 1.1, set within the context of professional practice.

Similarly, there are other concepts, shown in Figure 1.2, which will inform these interlocking ones, and these form the basis and structure of this book.

This first chapter sets the scene of professional development, exploring it within the context of expectations of professional practice and behaviour today, and within the educational philosophies of lifelong and continuous learning. With the development of nursing as a profession, and the fundamental changes within the National Health Service in Britain since the New Labour Government was elected in 1997, the need for continuous professional development, and accountability for practice has never been so apparent. Nurses are now expected to know more, do more, and take on more complicated and

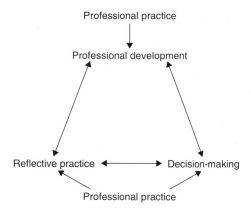

Figure 1.1 Links between professional development, reflective practice and decision-making.

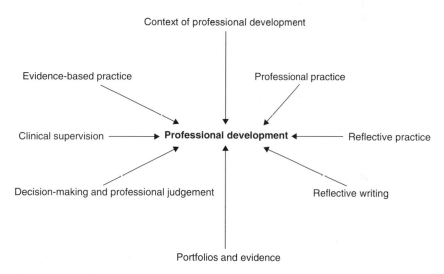

Figure 1.2 Concepts informing professional development.

expanding roles then ever before. With these comes greater independence and responsibility for their practice and for the service users within their care. This has brought concomitant changes in the regulatory processes, with the Nursing and Midwifery Council replacing the United Kingdom Central Council for Nursing, Midwifery and Health Visiting (UKCC) in 2002 and charged explicitly with 'protecting the public through professional standards'.

This chapter explores the processes of professional development that nurses go through – from being a novice student, through to the end of a career and working life in nursing. Whilst students and qualified practitioners undoubtedly face different challenges in their working lives, there are commonalities within the processes of professional development that apply across the experience divide. Balances need to be achieved between the external drivers for professional development – such as the need for a registerable qualification, for the development of recognised knowledge and skills, and for the demonstration of approved standards of practice – and the need for the less tangible personal development of feeling competent and confident, constantly challenging and learning new things that inform practice, and making a tangible difference to patient care through good individual practice. This chapter therefore takes an overview of what is meant by professional development, setting it within the context of nursing practice today. It ends with the introduction of a simple strategy for guiding your own professional development – go there now if you want to get started straight away. This strategy is called the '5WH' cues and runs throughout the book, focused to the subject matter that is being presented.

Chapters 2 and 3 consider the role of reflective practice and reflective writing within decision-making and professional development. Reflective practice is considered to be the way in which professionals learn from their experiences, create practice theory and develop expertise. The benefits of functioning as reflective practitioners – learning from and responsive to the changing environment of practice – are explored, and strategies for developing as a reflective practitioner are discussed. Reflective writing has a chapter in its own right, as development as a practitioner is as dependent upon an overt awareness of learning from practice, as it is on practice itself. Reflective writing provides ways of accessing and recognising experiential learning, through the dynamic use of writing as a process of learning, whilst at the same time providing evidence of professional development that is documented and evidenced. Reflective writing is presented as a strategy for guiding professional development and this strategy is used throughout the book using question stems – the 5WH cues. A key concept that emerged from a study exploring experienced nurses' use of reflective writing in their portfolios (Jasper 1999) was that nurses wanted to provide evidence of their professional accountability as practitioners through demonstrating their professional development, personal development, critical thinking development and, finally, the resultant outcomes for practice that occurred. Hence, there is a need to develop reflective writing skills as part of your own professional development.

Chapter 4 considers different strategies for professional decision-making. Georgina Koubel draws attention to the nebulous nature of professional decision-making, discussing the issues that need to be considered rather than taking a prescriptive approach. This is not the place to find a review of decision-making models and approaches, but rather to understand the complex nature of decision-making that occurs in professional practice.

Chapter 5 articulates with Chapter 4 in exploring the evidence-based practice debate, and looks at how this informs nurses' decision-making in practice. Evidence-based practice is a relatively new concept, and comprises decision-making for patients based on both the best available evidence and expert clinical judgement arising from experience. However, this is a hotly debated issue in health care, where several views can be taken about the need for generalisable data to inform decisions, versus the skill and experience of the professional in making individual judgements about individual patients. Gary Rolfe neatly summarises what can seem to be a very confusing debate, and poses questions for you to consider when making up your own mind on the issues.

Chapter 6 builds on the previous chapters to consider how nurses can use portfolios and construct evidence to facilitate and demonstrate their professional development. Key to portfolio development is identification of the reason it is being constructed and the purpose it is intended to serve. The portfolio's structure, process and content are all seen to be dependent upon this, as are the strategies within it that demonstrate the practitioner's competence to practise. Various structural models are considered, and Jasper's model is returned to as an alternative way of organising a portfolio.

Chapter 7 considers the role of clinical supervision in professional development. It summarises the key features of the concept to provide an easily understandable, and useful, guide to the concepts of supervision. However and perhaps more importantly, Paul Elliott challenges the confused terminology and conceptual basis of clinical supervision, suggesting that some of its problems in use in practice arise from these confusions. He presents alternative terminology and focus, preferring instead to consider clinical supervision as a form of 'person-centred development' that has its roots in health psychology.

Chapter 8 concludes the book by setting professional development within the confines of professional practice. In this chapter I explore the *Nursing and Midwifery Council Code of Professional Conduct: Standards for Conduct, Performance and Ethics* (NMC 2004a), together with other documents provided by the NMC to guide practitioners in their everyday practice. In addition, I will explore issues such as accountability, confidentiality and informed consent, as well as looking at recent legislation that impacts on a practitioner's working life. This chapter emphasises that professional practice is interdependent with professional development as that very practice is constantly changing and requires knowledge and skills to be updated on a continual basis.

Summary

- This book considers professional development, reflection and decision-making within the context of professional nursing practice in Britain today.
- It introduces a strategy for decision-making in professional development that is used throughout the book.

Activity

Before going any further, explore your own understanding of professional development.

Why is professional development important?
Why do professionals need development?
What drives professional development?
What would you consider professional development in nursing to mean?

The context of professional development in Britain today

All professionals practise within certain boundaries imposed by the society and culture that licenses them and the professional ethos of the profession to which they belong. For nurses, the authority to practise once qualified comes from four sources:

- Government legislation
- the Nursing and Midwifery Council
- their employers
- their service users.

All of these have certain expectations of a person qualified to call themselves a nurse, and indeed lay down certain standards of behaviour and practice that all professionals are required to adhere to. Within these expectations is the requirement that a professional practitioner will continue with their professional development throughout their working life (NMC 2004b).

Governmental influences on continuing professional development

In 2001, the Government introduced a framework for lifelong learning in the British National Health Service, with the aim of equipping staff with the skills they need to:

- support changes and improvements in patient care
- take advantage of wider career opportunities
- realise their potential.

(Department of Health 2001)

In *Working Together, Learning Together* (Department of Health 2001) the idea of the NHS as a 'learning organisation' with a commitment to professional development for all grades of staff was floated, with the aim of creating 'an organisation which puts lifelong learning at the heart of improving patient care'. In presenting the framework, the Government outlined their beliefs:

- a set of core values central to lifelong learning in the NHS and health care generally
- an entitlement to work in an environment which equips them with the skills to perform their current jobs to the best of their ability, developing their roles and career potential, working individually and in teams in more creative and fulfilling ways
- access to education, training and development should be as open and flexible as possible – with no discrimination in terms of age, gender, ethnicity
- learning should be valued, recognised, recorded and accredited wherever possible
- wherever practical, learning should be shared by different staff groups and professions
- planning and evaluation of lifelong learning should be central to organisational development and improvement, backed up by robust information about skills gaps and needs
- the infrastructure to support learning should be as close to the individual's workplace as possible, drawing on new educational and communications technology and designed to be accessible in terms of time and location.

(Department of Health 2001 p. 6)

This provides a framework for continuing professional development (CPD) for all staff, from the beginning student to the experienced practitioner. Student practitioner preparation is perceived as a partnership between the NHS and universities, with a 50:50 ratio between the time spent in practice placements and in the educational environment for nurses and midwives. Much CPD activity is commissioned by the NHS from universities, where strict quality assurance processes are imposed, both internally and externally, to ensure that educational activity is of high quality, appropriate for the NHS's needs and relevant for the individual practitioner. The Government further suggest that there are core knowledge and skills which should be common to all NHS employees. These are presented in Box 1.1.

With relevance for continuing professional development there is a requirement for the practitioner to:

'Demonstrate a commitment to keeping their skills and competence up to date – including the use of new apporaches to learning and using information – and supporting the learning and development of others.'
(Department of Health 2001 p. 8)

Box 1.1   Knowledge and Skills Framework: core knowledge and skills (Department of Health 2001 p. 7). Crown copyright is reproduced with the permission of the Controller of HMSO and the Queen's Printer for Scotland.

All staff should:

- fully understand and respect the rights and feelings of patients and their families, seeking out and addressing their needs
- communicate effectively with patients, their families and carers, and with colleagues
- value information about, and for, patients, as a privileged resource, sharing and using this appropriately, according to the discretion and consent allowed by the patient and by means of the most effective technology
- understand and demonstrate how the NHS, and their local organisation works
- work effectively in teams, appreciating the roles of other staff and agencies in the care of patients
- demonstrate a commitment to keeping their skills and competence up to date, including the use of new approaches to learning
- using information and supporting the learning and development of others, recognise and demonstrate their responsibilities for maintaining the health and safety of patients and colleagues in all care settings.

This is reinforced by various other strategies and by the professional body. Within the current legislation there are three major initiatives which affect the professional development for all nurses and midwives:

- the introduction of personal development plans
- the Knowledge and Skills Framework
- the skills escalator approach.

These will each be considered in the following sections.

Summary

- Government legislation places a responsibility on all practitioners to engage in professional development.
- As the major health and social care employer, the NHS has a commitment to lifelong learning for all employees.
- Reform of the NHS has resulted in a focus on individual development alongside service delivery needs.

Personal development plans

Central to the notion of lifelong learning is for all employees to have *personal development plans*. These were first conceived in the publication *Continuous Professional Development: Quality in the NHS* (Department of

Health 2000) which recognised the potential for every individual to progress and develop throughout their working lives. *Working Together, Learning Together* (Department of Health 2001) identified personal development plans (PDPs) as the strategy by which all practitioners would identify and meet their short-term professional development needs.

The 'personal' in PDPs refers to the plan being individualised, but it is not intended to cover the personal areas of the practitioner's life. To this extent, they are really *professional* development plans, in that they are intended to help the practitioner plan and achieve their development throughout their career.

Interestingly, the idea of PDPs for students in higher education was introduced a few years earlier in the *Dearing Report* (NCIHE 1997) which recommended that all students would be using them by 2005/2006. Personal development planning is seen as:

> '*A structured and supported process undertaken by an individual to reflect upon their own learning, performance and/or achievement and to plan for their personal, educational and career development.*' (Universities UK, SCOP, Universities Scotland, LTSN, QAA 2001 p. 1)

As a result, the majority of student practitioners will now be familiar with PDPs and used to completing these as they progress through their programme of study. However, the nature of these may be somewhat different to those expected by employers of qualified staff.

First, for students, the PDP may be a private document that has to be completed but is not actually seen by anyone else. This may form the basis of discussion with academic staff, but the student cannot be required to show the work to anyone. This enables it to become the repository of incidents and reflective material for the student, without fear that it may be accessed by others. Second, parts of the PDP may be copied in a progress file, which is open for access to others and officially documents the student's route and achievements during their studies. Third, this use of PDPs helps the student gain the skills needed in planning their professional development and prepares them to take on the responsibility for their own PDP as a qualified practitioner.

For qualified staff, the nature of the PDP is likely to be very different in that it is a requirement by the employer and may be an entirely public document used in appraisals or job applications. Many practitioners are content to remain within the main career grades of nursing and midwifery; as a female dominated profession, this will often include periods of part-time or night-time working to accommodate family responsibilities and career breaks. However, whilst it is accepted that the majority of nurses work within nursing as a job, they do still have a responsibility as a professional to ensure that they remain competent and safe to practise, and that they are providing optimum care for their patients. Your employer may have certain elements of a PDP that they require you to complete on a regular basis to ensure that they are meeting their own targets for lifelong learning and staff development.

Personal development plans provide a way of continually engaging with your own professional development, even if it is not included within a larger professional portfolio. They are a useful developmental tool for enabling a practitioner to consider their developmental needs, and to plan how these can be achieved. They also act as a stimulus for reflective practice, and a strategy for the practitioner to use to review their practice over time.

Summary

- Every student and NHS employee will need to have a personal development plan.
- Students use them as part of their study programme, to document their progress and to plan for their educational needs.
- Students' PDPs are usually private and not seen by others.
- Qualified practitioners working in the NHS can use PDPs for their own individual plans for development.
- Many employers now use PDPs within their appraisal strategy, to enable practitioners to work with their managers to plan and achieve their own professional development.
- These are, essentially therefore, public documents that are required as a condition of employment.

Activity

If you do not already use a PDP, consider the following:

What would you use a PDP for?
Do you need to have one?
Do you need to find out more about them?

The Knowledge and Skills Framework

> 'The Knowledge and Skills Framework describes and defines the knowledge and skills which the NHS staff need to apply in their work to deliver quality services. It provides a single, consistent, comprehensive and explicit framework on which to base review and development for all staff.' (Department of Health 2004 p. 3)

This framework is being used to drive the reform of the career and pay progression structures within the NHS, and involves a developmental review process. It is one of the three components of *Agenda for Change* (HSC 227 1999) together with job evaluation, and terms and conditions. The purpose of the KSF is to:

- facilitate the development of services so that they better meet the needs of users and the public through investing in the development of all members of staff
- support the effective learning and development of individuals and teams
- support the development of individuals in the post in which they are employed so that they can be effective at work
- promote equality and diversity of all staff.

(Adapted from Department of Health 2004 p. 4)

The intention is that the KSF will apply to all members of staff (except doctors, dentists, senior managers and board level) because it is intended to be:

- NHS wide
- developed and implemented in partnership
- developmental
- equitable
- simple and feasible to implement
- capable of linking with current and emerging competence frameworks (such as national occupational standards and QAA benchmarks).

The KSF focuses on the *application* of knowledge, rather than the specific knowledge and skills that people need to develop. This knowledge is related to what is needed by a person in order to meet the demands of their job. The KSF is made up of 30 dimensions, six of which are *core* dimensions:

(1) communication
(2) personal and people development
(3) health, safety and security
(4) service improvement
(5) quality
(6) equality and diversity.

These dimensions identify the broad functions required by the NHS to enable it to provide a good-quality service for the public. The other dimensions are more specific, and apply to some, but not all jobs in the NHS. They are grouped into the themes and are listed in Table 1.1:

- health and well-being
- estates and facilities
- information and knowledge
- general.

Table 1.1 Specific themes of the *Knowledge and Skills Framework*.

Health and well-being	General
Promotion of health and well-being and prevention of adverse effects to health and well-being Assessment and care planning to meet health and well-being needs Protection of health and well-being Enablement to address health and well-being needs Provision of care to meet health and well-being needs Assessment and treatment planning Interventions and treatments Biomedical investigation and intervention Equipment and devices to meet health and well-being needs Products to meet health and well-being needs	Learning and development Development and innovation Procurement and commissioning Financial management Services and project management People management Capacity and capability Public relations and marketing
Estates and facilities	**Information and knowledge**
Systems, vehicles and equipment Environments and buildings Transport and logistics	Information processing Information collection and analysis Knowledge and information sources

Source: Department of Health 2001 pp. 6–7.

Each dimension has four levels, which describe and indicate how the knowledge and skills need to be applied at that level. This means that for the individual practitioner to achieve a certain level they need to be able to show that they can apply knowledge and skills to meet all of the indicators at that level. These are shown for the core dimensions in Table 1.2.

All posts in the NHS will be evaluated against the *Knowledge and Skills Framework*. This provides the professional practitioner with a useful indication of what knowledge and skills they will need in order to be able to progress in their career. As a result, they can use this to plan their own professional development.

Summary

- *The Knowledge and Skills Framework* defines the knowledge and skills framework required for different posts in the NHS.
- All jobs will be evaluated against the framework.
- The framework contains 30 dimensions.
- Six of these are core dimensions and apply to every job: communication; personal and people development; health, safety and security; service improvement; quality; and equality and diversity.
- The other dimensions only apply to certain jobs.

Table 1.2 Indicators of the core dimensions of the *Knowlege and Skills Framework.*

Dimensions	Level descriptors			
CORE	1	2	3	4
1 Communication	Communicate with a limited range of people on a day-to-day basis	Communicate with a range of people on a range of matters	Develop and maintain communication with people about difficult matters and/or in difficult situatons	Develop and maintain communication with people on complex matters, issues and ideas and/or in complex situations
2 Personal and people development	Contribute to own personal development	Develop own skills and knowledge and provide information to others to help their development	Develop oneself and contribute to the development of others	Develop oneself and others in areas of practice
3 Health, safety and security	Assist in maintaining own and others' health, safety and security	Monitor and maintain health, safety and security of self and others	Promote, monitor and maintain best practice in health, safety and security	Maintain and develop an environment and culture that improves health, safety and security
4 Service improvement	Make changes in own practice and offer suggestions for improving services	Contribute to the improvement of services	Appraise, interpret and apply suggestions, recommendations and directives to improve services	Work in partnership with others to develop, take forward and evaluate direction, policies and strategies
5 Quality	Maintain the quality of own work	Maintain quality in own work and encourage others to do so	Contribute to improving quality	Develop a culture that improves quality
6 Equality and diversity	Act in ways that support equality and value diversity	Support equality and value diversity	Promote equality and value diversity	Develop a culture that promotes equality and values diversity

Source: Department of Health 2001 p. 8. Crown copyright is reproduced with the permission of the Controller of HMSO and the Queen's Printer for Scotland.

- The KSF can be used to plan a practitioner's professional development by comparing present knowledge and skills with those expected at the next career point.

The skills escalator approach

Working Together, Learning Together (Department of Health 2001 p. 17) introduced the *skills escalator* as an approach to supporting staff in progressing through their careers. It recognises that care delivery in the NHS is not only delivered by those with a professional qualification, but is supported by many who work in 'diverse and important jobs, all of which are integral to modernising care and service delivery'. These include health care assistants, medical secretaries, IT mechanics, porters, laboratory technicians, to name but a few. The skills escalator is designed to move people up a skills development programme. Table 1.3 illustrates the skills escalator approach.

As a result of the recognition of the educational and learning needs for all grades and types of staff in the NHS, we have seen the widening and development of opportunities for learning from school and college level qualifications, to professional and post-qualifying programmes as described in the skills escalator. This has provided a route for professional development through career development, whilst recognising that many members of staff are content to remain in their grade and still need developmental opportunities throughout their working lives.

Summary

- The skills escalator approach defines career progression through the NHS for all employees.
- It enables professional practitioners to plan their professional development if they want to go up the career ladder.

Activity

How can the KSF and skills escalator help you in planning your own career progression and professional development activity?

Consider the elements of each one, and use these to identify your professional development needs.

The role of the Nursing and Midwifery Council

The Nursing and Midwifery Council was established in 2002 as the regulatory body for nurses, midwives and specialist community public health nurses[1], with the purpose of establishing and improving stan-

---

[1] The term Health Visitor was replaced by the term Specialist Community Public Health Nurse with the creation of the third part of the nurses and midwives register in 2004.

Table 1.3 The skills escalator approach.

Category	Means of career progression
Socially excluded individuals with difficulties in obtaining employment ↓	Six-month employment orientation programmes to develop basic understanding of the world of work
The unemployed ↓	Six-month placements in 'starter' jobs, rotating into different areas of work, whilst undertaking structured training and development
Jobs/roles requiring fewer skills and less experience, e.g. cleaning, catering, portering ↓	Skills modules to support progression through job rotation and development programmes including NVQs and NHS learning agreements, appraisal and personal development planning
Skilled roles, e.g. health care assistants. Other support staff ↓	Modules of training and development through NVQs or equivalent vocational qualifications
Qualified professional staff, e.g. nurses, therapists, scientists, junior managers ↓	First jobs/roles following formal pre-registration education or conversion courses. Appraisal and personal development planning to support career progression. Achievement of a range of skills acquired at staged intervals
More advanced skills and roles, e.g. expert practitioners, middle managers, training and non-medical role/grades ↓	Further progression, supported and demonstrated through learning and skills development as above. Flexible working and role development encouraged in line with service priorities and personal career choices
'Consultant' roles, e.g. clinical and scientific professionals, senior managers	Flexible 'portfolio careers' for newly appointed, experienced and supervising roles, planned in partnership with employers informed by robust appraisal, career and PDP processes

Source: Department of Health 2001 p. 18. Crown copyright is reproduced with the permission of the Controller of HMSO and the Queen's Printer for Scotland.

dards of care in order to serve and protect the public. It replaced the previous body, the United Kingdom Council for Nurses, Midwives and Health Visitors. Its key tasks are to:

- maintain a register of qualified nurses, midwives and specialist community public health nurses
- set standards and guidelines for education, practice and conduct
- provide advice on professional standards

- consider allegations of misconduct or unfitness to practise due to ill health. (NMC 2004a)

Student nurses and midwives are expected to acquire these attributes of professional practice as they progress through their initial pro-gramme of study. Hence, their professional development commences as soon as they begin their course. Upon qualification, all nurses and midwives are accountable to the NMC for their practice, and for demonstrating their competence to practise under the Post-Registration Education and Practice (PREP) standards.

In 2004 the NMC re-issued *The PREP Handbook* (2004b), which out-lines the requirements for continuing professional development and practice established by its predecessor, the United Kingdom Central Council for Nursing, Midwifery and Health Visiting. These are:

- **The PREP (practice) standard:** you must have worked in some capacity by virtue of your nursing or midwifery qualification during the previous five years for a minimum of 100 days (750 hours), or have successfully undertaken an approved return to practice course.
- **The PREP (continuing professional development) standard:** you must have undertaken and recorded your continuing professional development (CPD) over the three years prior to the renewal of your registration. All registered nurses and midwives have been required to comply with this standard since April 1995. Since April 2000, registrants need to have declared on their notification to prac-tise form that they have met this requirement when they renew their registration. (NMC 2004b pp. 4–5)

The PREP (CPD) standard is further explained as a need to:

- undertake at least five days or 35 hours of learning activity relevant to your practice during the three years prior to your renewal of registration
- maintain a personal professional profile (PPP) of your learning
- comply with any request from the NMC to audit how you have met these requirements. (NMC 2004b p. 7)

Activity

Have you complied with the PREP standards in the past three years?
How have you recorded this?
What evidence do you have that would prove this to another person?

The NMC goes on to emphasise that the learning undertaken must be relevant to your practice, but there is no such thing as an approved learning activity. This provides the practitioner with considerable scope in choosing what they consider is appropriate to demonstrate the CPD standard. They also say that 'you must document, in your PPP, your relevant learning activity and the way in which it has informed and influenced your practice'. The NMC do not expect the PPP to be presented in an approved format, so, again, this is left to the discretion of the practitioner. They do, though, provide a template for recording this activity that can be used (this will be discussed in Chapter 6).

Professional development, then, is seen as a continuous process that starts as a student and carries on for the whole of a practitioner's working life. During this time, students learn what it is to be a professional practitioner and become socialised into how that profession carries out its business. Entry to the profession is judged on the basis of fitness to practise, or competence, measured against criteria specified by the NMC. They also specify criteria for ongoing competence and safe practice, providing a framework within which anyone wanting to practise as a registered nurse or midwife must locate their practice.

Summary

- Professional development starts as a student and carries on throughout a practitioner's working life.
- All nurses and midwives must achieve the PREP practice and CPD standards in order to re-register every three years.
- It doesn't have to cost you any money.
- There is no such thing as approved PREP (CPD) learning activity.
- You don't need to collect points or certificates of attendance.
- There is no approved format for the personal professional profile.
- It must be relevant to the work you are doing and/or plan to do in the near future.
- It must help you to provide the highest possible standards of care for your patients and clients.

Expectations of your employers

Your employer is contracted to provide a service to others that delivers to a standard that has previously been agreed by the parties involved in the contract. As an employee of the NHS, or even of independent health care providers, the standards of this service are negotiated by others on behalf of the service user, and you are expected to achieve this standard. Your employer therefore has a vested interest in the competence of the staff they employ, and a need to ensure adequate professional development for its practitioners. They can require you to undergo professional development as part of your employment.

Much of the responsibility for professional development comes in the form of devolved responsibility from Government policy, such as through the *Knowledge and Skills Framework*, and through target setting. The Nursing and Midwifery Council also lays specific responsibilities on employers, such as checking the qualifications and currency of registration of applicants for posts, and in expecting contraventions of the code of professional conduct to be reported to the Fitness to Practice committee. Your employer is expected to ensure that all employees achieve minimum standards of ongoing development, such as mandatory training in fire safety and manual handling, for instance, as well as providing opportunities for professional education that enable practitioners to achieve the CPD requirements of their profession. Most employers go beyond these basics of course, and use education budgets to support individuals through further education and qualifications in order for them to be able to work in different or new roles, or have career progression.

However, whilst most employers do support their staff in achieving the minimum CPD standards, it is the *responsibility* of the registrant (practitioner) to ensure that they comply with the standard; the practitioner cannot claim that their employer did not enable them to comply by not giving them time off for study. As a professional you are expected to ensure you comply with this standard.

Summary

- Employers have a duty to ensure their employees are competent to do the job they are employed to do.
- They can require you to engage in professional development as part of your employment.
- Engaging in achieving the minimum CPD standard for registration is the responsibility of the practitioner.

Service user expectations

Finally, service users invest in practitioners a belief that they will care for them competently and to the best of their ability. They trust you to recognise the limits of your knowledge, skills and experience and to treat them appropriately. Relationships between service users and professional practitioners, although subject to many written rules (such as the code of professional conduct, informed consent etc.) are usually tacit, unspoken agreements that both parties have an understanding of, and respect the boundaries within which they operate.

For instance, much professional practice involves the practitioner in touching the body of their patients. The patient is usually a stranger, and under normal circumstances one person would not touch a stranger unless invited to do so. In the practitioner–patient relationship the 'rules' of touching are different, in that the practitioner may touch (or examine) the part of the patient that is causing a problem, or may access other parts of the person for diagnosis and treatment. However, these parameters are tightly construed by both sides, even if unwittingly and subconsciously. On the whole, the majority of 'touching' relationships overcome feelings of embarrassment because they remain within the expected parameters. However, at times, these boundaries may be overstepped, and touching happens that is considered inappropriate; this may be in the place that a patient is touched, or the nature of touching. This may lead to accusations of professional misconduct, or criminal prosecutions.

Another area where service users implicitly trust practitioners is in the belief or title, uniforms and qualifications – the overt manifestations of power. Professionals and service users are in an unequal relationship because the professionals usually possess more knowledge about a patient's condition than the patient. This is being addressed in schemes such as the Expert Patient Scheme, the use of service users' representatives at all levels in the NHS, and the increasing recognition by professionals that patients are partners in care as opposed to being passive recipients of it. Patients have trust in professionals because they have expectations of what the titles and uniforms mean. They take professional advice because it comes from a professional, whom they believe to have the appropriate knowledge and understanding to be able to provide that advice.

In terms of professional development, then, as practitioners we are responsible to our service users to ensure that we are providing the best possible care and advice to them that we are able to give. To some extent this means updating our knowledge and basing practice on the best, and most relevant, evidence available; admitting our limitations and rectifying these and ensuring that we are competent to practice.

Summary

- Service users have a right to expect a high-quality standard of care from professional practitioners.
- The service user–practitioner relationship is a special one based on trust and respect, and enables the practitioner to access both the physical and personal space of the service user.
- This is permitted because the service user believes the practitioner will deliver the best advice and care that they can.
- The practitioner therefore has a duty to maintaining their CPD for the sake of their service users.

Professional development activities

Anything that you do that contributes to your own knowledge base, understanding and skill can be seen as professional development.

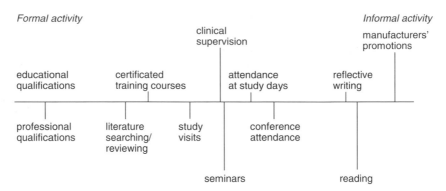

Figure 1.3 Professional development activities.

Perhaps the most important criteria are that you recognise that you are developing and changing as a result of your activities. Professional development activities can be seen as a continuum, with formal academic qualifications at one extreme, and personal individual reflective activity at the other. I have presented this continuum in Figure 1.3. The order of these activities on the formal–informal line is of course arbitrary, but this will help, I hope, to provide some idea of the range of activities that you may use.

Activity

How many of these activities have you engaged in over the past three years?
Have you done anything else, that isn't in this list?
What records do you have of these activities?
How have you used the learning from them to inform your practice?

Formal professional development activities will, of necessity, provide evidence of your professional development. Any assessments that you complete will be in a written format that creates a permanent record. Similarly, attendance at study days, mandatory training activities, or conferences will also provide you with permanent evidence. The further across the continuum you go towards informal and unstructured activities, the less likely you are to have ready-made evidence of your developmental activities. To some extent, at a personal level, this may not matter. However, all nurses and midwives registered on the live professional register maintained by the Nursing and Midwifery Council need to provide evidence of their continuing professional development in order to re-register every three years. This means that you will need to find ways of recording your activities and creating evidence if you wish informal learning and development to count towards your CPD standard. You may choose to do this through reflective reviews, commentaries and writing; strategies for doing this will be explored in more detail in Chapter 3. You may choose to use a professional portfolio to accumulate a continuous record of your development; strategies for portfolio development will be explored in Chapter 6. Portfolios can accommodate a range of evidence and activities, and this will be the place to write up work, such as searching literature, reflecting on learning from clinical supervision, or critical incident analysis amongst other things.

A model of professional development

In 1984, Patricia Benner published her work on professional development, or skills acquisition, entitled *From Novice to Expert*. Benner, drawing on the work of Dreyfus and Dreyfus (1986) identified five stages through which she considered nurses pass in moving from being a new recruit to the profession to reaching expertise as a practitioner. This work provided the profession with much food for thought in considering how nurses move from being students through to advanced practice in an incremental way, identifying key features of how they practise during this transition. Benner suggested that, in addition to displaying certain attributes of practice at each of these stages, a nurse needed to spend a defined number of years within each stage before hoping to be considered to have moved to the next stage. This feature of her model has been disputed and is now largely discounted by those who use the model, who consider that educational development and processes can outweigh or override the need to spend a specified amount of time in a practice environment.

Another feature of Benner's model was the notion of transferability of the stages of skills acquisition between different clinical environments. For example, a nurse who is considered an expert in neonatal baby care would not be considered an expert if she went to work on a unit caring for elderly patients suffering from dementia. Whilst there is some logic to this argument, several authors have suggested that transferable skills are utilised in any area of practice, and that whilst the specifics of practice relating to the client group may not be at expert level, other ways of practising, such as the thought processes used, will still be utilised.

Robinson *et al.* (2003) translated Benner's stages of development into a model that related to the qualified nursing working force in an American hospital. They combined two of Benner's stages (novice and advanced beginner) as they found the distinction between the two in relation to qualified staff unclear, then applied the model to a classification of their nursing staff. This model enables nursing management to assess nurses' skills and attributes and identify professional development needs within the organisation. Table 1.4 shows the features of

Table 1.4 A model of professional development.

The novice practitioner	The competent practitioner	The proficient practitioner	The expert practitioner
• is new to nursing practices from a theoretical knowledge base while recognising and providing for routine patient needs • is beginning to incorporate his/her theoretical knowledge into clinical situations and is able to perform basic skills and carry out a plan of care • can identify abnormal findings, but may seek consultation for solutions • practice is primarily guided by policies, procedures, and standards • words/phrases in the job description for the RN 1 include basic, uncomplicated, seeks appropriate information, and may require assistance • however, the expectation was advancement to the next level of practice within 1 year • this category encompasses student nurses	• in Britain, is the point of qualification • has mastered the technical skills • is aware of patterns of patient responses and can use past experiences to identify solutions for current situations • focuses on outcomes • patients and families are incorporated into the clinical focus • care is delivered using a systematic practitioner approach • is able to make independent decisions guided by experience as well as policies and standards • continues to consult other members of the health care team when the need for assistance is identified • key words/phrases that define this nurse include	• has an in-depth knowledge of nursing practice • relies on previous experience for focused analysis of problems and solutions • recognises situations as a whole • he/she can accommodate unplanned events and respond with speed, efficiency, flexibility, and confidence • views patients holistically with an integrated, collaborative approach to care • uses standards of practice as guidelines with individual patient modification in order to meet outcomes • is beginning to assume a leadership role within the clinical practice area, using expertise to serve as a role model, preceptor, and coach • in the job	• functions from an intuitive base • has developed a comprehensive knowledge base • is self-directed, flexible and innovative in providing patient care • operates from a deep understanding of a total situation to resolve complex issues • works collaboratively with the other health care team providers to support the patient/family in achieving goals • actively and positively influences the team, fosters critical thinking in others, and forms mentoring relationships with other nurses • participates and leads activities that improve systems for quality patient care • serves as a change agent to challenge themselves and others • words used to define this nurse include expertly, initiates, mentors and leads • approximately 5% of staff nurses are expected to fulfil the requirements for the expert nurse

Table 1.4 *Continued*

The novice practitioner	The competent practitioner	The proficient practitioner	The expert practitioner
	consistent, independent, able to individualise care and prioritises care activities • at this level of practice, the nurse can comfortably care for any patient in the clinical area • the majority of nurses (60%) in the organisation are expected to be in this category	description this nurse is described by words and phrases such as anticipates, critically analyses, is a role model, and resource person • approximately 20% of nurses in the organisation will be in this category	

Source: adapted from Benner (1984) and Robinson *et al.* (2003) to reflect nursing in Britain.

nurses at these different stages, adapted from the work of both Benner and Robinson *et al.*

Activity

Looking at these key features of each stage, whereabouts would you consider your practice to be?
Why?
Is this where you would like your practice to be, or would you like to move into another category?
What would you need to do to be able to do this?

In a British context, this is a useful model to identify the process of professional development (seeing the student as a novice) through the career path of a nurse to advanced or expert practice. Neither Benner nor Robinson *et al.* considered that all practitioners would progress to the final stage of expert practice. Benner saw this as being achieved only after 5–7 years of practice in a particular environment, and accompanied by specific ways of practice that separated the proficient practitioner from the expert. Similarly, Robinson *et al.* estimated that only 5% of their staff would achieve expert practice. This equates well with the British situation, in that whilst we have had specialist nurses developing their practice in focused ways for some time, we now have a tier of modern matrons and consultants who are all expected to be functioning above the specialist level, and to achieve independence in their practice over and above what has previously been recognised. This is not to say that we did not have expert nurses in the past, but rather that we now have mechanisms to recognise and reward these nurses, whilst at the same time maximising their potential within an organisation.

The novice practitioner

The novice is generally new to nursing. In Britain, we expect the novice to gain knowledge, experience and skills throughout their pre-registration education to enable them to enter the profession on graduation as competent practitioners. Students in Britain spend half their programme in clinical practice working within a partnership model of education that gives joint responsibility for the standards that students achieve in practice to both the educational institution and the health authority where they work. This differs from the American model where the student has little exposure to the real world of nursing practice during their initial preparation and is considered a novice for the first year, at least, of qualified practice.

As a novice practitioner, the student nurse is dependent on learning the rules that govern that practice and acquiring a body of knowledge that enables them to understand the guiding principles behind what they are doing. The novice practitioner is therefore quite slow in what they do, as they need to think about what they do at all times and follow procedural steps in giving care. Little that they do is based on experience of the situation, and in assessing patients' needs and devising care plans they will be dependent on established routines and practices arising from what they see others doing. They need to be safe in what they are doing and therefore defer to other nurses' knowledge and experiences, and will be working in a supervised capacity. They can identify abnormal findings because their theoretical parameters are more advanced than their practice ones, but may seek consultation for solutions.

Student nurses have a minimum of three years to move from novice to competent practice, and at some point in this time pass through what Benner called the 'advanced beginner' stage.

Many authors have studied the transition of student nurses into qualified practitioners, and identify a transformational confusion that accompanies the change in status from being a student to having one's own responsibility as a nurse. Jenny Spouse (2003) studied a group of student nurses throughout their three-year training programme and identified the process of professional development that students go through in order to take on the characteristics of a qualified nurse. This is essentially a socialisation process, as the student acquires the beliefs and values, knowledge and skills, and social attributes of what is expected of a nurse. Spouse suggests that this involves four components:

- **Social aspects:** these are the existing customs and practices that maintain the profession's homogeneity and create a shared identity. Students have a choice in whether to conform and adopt these norms and thus be accepted, or whether to resist these and be rejected by the profession.
- **Identity and evolving self-image as a member of the community:** the student needs to look and act like a professional nurse, adopting behaviour, language, dress and modes of thought that characterise the community. This enables the status quo to be maintained and facilitates teamworking. Spouse found that students who brought with them a strong sense of 'ideal practice', or what it is to be a 'good' nurse, were able to adapt to what they met in practice, and adopt acceptable behaviours as they were able to match what they saw happening against their beginning beliefs and values, and standards of expectations of practice. Fitting into the clinical situation is key for the student's progress and acceptance by the nursing team as this influences the learning opportunities available to them and the ways in which others will relate to them during their time in placement.
- **Role acquisition:** the student has an anxiety to do well and is preoccupied with 'fitting in'. Key to this is the quality of relationships with clinical staff; this enables effective role modelling to occur and assists the student to learn the cultural norms of each placement. Whilst these may differ between placements, they gradually build up to provide a set of working practices that are acceptable and approved within the organisation, so that once the student qualifies he/she is able to fit into the working environment of that particular organisation. Many universities now allocate students to 'home trusts', learning communities or ward bases, where they spend the majority of their clinical time. If they live locally, these placements are likely to be in the organisation where they will gain their first job as a qualified nurse. This helps them to move more comfortably into the qualified nurse role as they already have familiarity with the culture existent in that organisation, and are

also likely to have worked in the environment as a student. Students need, according to Benner (1984), to build 'a repertoire of paradigm cases' by exposure to a wide range of clinical and patient situations. These form the basis of experiential learning, whereby the student mentally stores these cases and subconsciously draws on them each time a similar event occurs. In this way the student builds up their experience, and through reflective learning processes can use them as learning experiences. Hence, the student needs to be accepted into the clinical team and provided with as wide a range of experience as possible to help them achieve their learning objectives and thus become a nurse. In acquiring this role identity students become like the role models they see around them, for example an adult, children's or mental health nurse, and 'feel' like them. In many ways this reinforces their commitment to their chosen field of nursing and gives them enormous pleasure as they fit in with the other practitioners around them and are accepted as 'one of them'.

- **Feeling and acting like a nurse:** finally, the student has acquired sufficient professional characteristics to have a 'personal construct' as a nurse, which enables them to act like a nurse and be acceptable to their professional colleagues. Students who adopt these characteristics incompletely, or fail to transform into these professional expectations, find it difficult to adjust to professional practice and may be ambivalent about staying in the profession, or uncomfortable with their role (Spouse 2003). Spouse suggests that the students need to adopt one or more personalities and roles defined by the different environments in which they work (academic, professional and social) in order to achieve an equilibrium they can cope with. If the student cannot adapt to this, again, they may leave the profession.

In learning to be a professional, Spouse (2003) suggests that the novice practitioner needs to acquire several specific areas of practice competence:

- relating to patients and their carers
- developing technical knowledge
- learning to bundle nursing activities together
- developing craft knowledge
- managing feelings and emotions
- developing the essence of nursing which promotes therapeutic action
- relating to and functioning within a clinical team.

These are in addition to developing a professional knowledge base that underpins all practice elements.

Activity

The specific areas of practice competence identified by Spouse provide a useful framework for identifying our own progress and development, especially if used within a reflective framework and/or a portfolio of skills acquisition. Take some time to consider your own competence in these areas by making a table of them and writing down, against each one, some examples of your skill in them.

There are several ways that students can learn to use the resources available to them in the clinical environment in order to maximise their learning opportunities:

- understanding your role as a student
- creating a personal development plan, that gives you clear objectives and ways of achieving these
- using key informants in the clinical setting
- developing a clear student–mentor relationship
- expecting good mentoring
- focusing on your learning needs
- making the most of opportunities available to you
- being flexible in your working hours to ensure you are around when things happen
- making the most of your supernumerary status.

Professional development for a student is about learning to be a safe and competent practitioner who has sufficient knowledge and skills to be fit for the purpose for which they are employed. These foundations lay the base for professional practice and development by enabling them to work effectively and knowledgeably within a clinical environment as well as having generic attitudes and transferable skills on which they can build their working lives. Becoming a professional involves more than just learning the theory and practice of nursing; it includes taking on professional attributes and characteristics that mark you out as a member of the nursing profession, such as:

- interpersonal communication skills
- working as a member of a team
- being responsible for your own professional development
- updating your evidence base for practice
- developing your powers of critical thinking
- developing the skills of a reflective practitioner.

Summary

- Students are novice practitioners who need to adopt rule-bound behaviours to be safe in their practice.

- Professional development for student nurses involves learning the attributes of being a professional through socialisation processes.
- Novice practitioners work through the advanced beginner stage to become competent by acquiring the knowledge base, skills and experience in order to be fit for practice on qualification.
- Professional development involves more than acquiring a theoretical knowledge base and skills; it also involves ways of communicating and acting that mark you out as a member of a profession.

The competent nurse

The competent nurse is one who has mastered sufficient technical skills to be aware of patterns of patient responses and can draw on past experiences, as well as policies and procedures, to inform any current situations they are faced with, thus enabling them to be accountable and responsible for their practice. This individualised practice is set within the environment of inter-professional and mono-professional teamwork, as the competent nurse is keenly aware of his/her role within the team and limitations of his/her own practice. This provides safety for the practitioner as they know they can consult with others and draw on the vast range of experience available within their work environment. Robinson *et al.* (2003) saw 60% of the staff in their organisation as being at this level, providing significant challenges for professional development to enable them to move to more proficient practice where they were able to accept higher levels of independence and responsibility.

Competent nurses may build a wealth of experience within the clinical environment, and consider themselves to be experts in this care over a number of years. Yet, often this view of themselves is based on length of time and familiarity rather than as a result of professional development that can be equated with incremental knowledge and skills development, and an awareness of their own learning and growth as practitioners. Custom and practice can result in stagnation if a nurse does not see a need to question their own practice. Hence, every practitioner needs to have their own personal development plan, either separate from or as part of their professional portfolio, which helps them to learn and move their practice forward continually.

Summary

- Competent nurses are confident in their knowledge, skills and abilities to provide patient care.
- They make up the majority of the nursing workforce.
- Professional development activities need to be focused on ensuring evidence-based and up-to-date practice.

The proficient nurse

Proficient nurses have an in-depth knowledge of nursing practice as a result of the time and experience they have built up in a specific clinical area. They rely on this previous experience to guide their problem-solving and decision-making, and for focused analysis of problems and solutions. This differs from the modes of practice identified at the previous two stages, which depend more on the overt use of rules and theoretical perspectives to inform practice. At the proficient stage, knowledge and experience are integrated into a whole, and all sources of information are drawn upon in an intuitive way. Situations themselves are recognised and reacted to as a whole. A bank of experience, called 'paradigm cases' by Benner, enables the practitioner to accommodate unplanned events and respond with speed, efficiency, flexibility, and confidence because they do not have to stop to consciously work out and think through courses of action. Similarly, patients are viewed holistically as individuals, with an integrated, collaborative approach to care taken to ensure the most appropriate care package is devised and delivered. Standards of practice are used as guidelines only – decisions are made on the basis of evidence-based practice using the best available evidence combined with clinical judgement, resulting in individual patient modification to treatment regimes in order to meet outcomes. This practitioner is beginning, or has been promoted, to assume a leadership role within the clinical practice area, using expertise to serve as a role model, preceptor and coach. Their practice is characterised by higher level cognitive skills such as anticipation of patient events and predicting patterns and outcomes; critically analysing clinical situations and looking for alternative courses of action; being broad and open-minded; being a role model and resource person for others in the profession. The proficient nurse is most likely to be in a care management role, such as ward or clinical manager, or acting in a specialist role following years of experience in the specialty. Benner considered that proficiency followed competency as a result of experience and development within that particular area. Robinson *et al.* suggest that approximately 20% of nurses in an organisation will be at the proficient stage.

Proficient nurses usually have career expectations to move beyond the main nursing grades. They often aspire to independent or advanced practice, and therefore tend to be self-sufficient in their professional development by taking the initiative and fulfilling their own developmental needs.

Summary

- Proficient nurses act in a beginning leadership capacity.
- They are likely to have considerable specialist knowledge and may act as nurse specialists.

- Proficient nurses often aspire to career progression.
- Professional development activity is focused on achieving higher levels of knowledge and skill for future practice roles.

The expert nurse

The expert nurse or advanced practitioner functions from an intuitive base and has developed a comprehensive knowledge base through years of experience combined with continuous professional development activities. As a result, the expert practitioner can function independently, being self-directed, flexible and innovative in providing patient care. As complex and critical thinkers, experts are reflective practitioners who operate from a deep understanding of a total situation to resolve complex issues in the absence of complete information. Although capable of independent practice, the expert works collaboratively with the inter-professional team where needed to ensure that the patient is always the focus of health care delivery. The expert nurse takes an equal place in the multi-professional team, actively and positively influencing the team, fostering critical thinking in others, and forming mentoring relationships with other nurses. They take a leadership role in their own specialist area of practice, exploring and researching care strategies as well as leading practice development. Therefore, expert nurses act as change agents to move practice forward and contribute to knowledge creation in their field. The role components adopted by expert practitioners may include:

- mentorship
- leadership
- being seen as a role model
- acting as a source of authority
- acting as a change agent
- influencing policy and practice development
- acting as an expert witness.

In Britain, the Government created Nurse Consultant posts (Department of Health 1999) which have four core functions:

- expert practice
- professional leadership and consultancy
- education and development
- practice and service development.

Consultant nurses are expected to be those practitioners at the leading and cutting edge of their speciality, and to retain a clinical component to their role where they continue to practise their speciality. The Royal College of Nursing, in Britain, through the work of the Practice Development Unit, has helped to frame and develop the concept of the consultant nurse through the work of Kim Manley and her colleagues.

Manley (1997) suggests that in addition to the components identified by the Government, consultant nurses need to be:

- researchers with experience in practice-based methodologies
- expert and process consultants from clinical to executive and strategic levels
- transformational leaders.

This has been groundbreaking work that has enabled nurses to achieve career progression beyond the traditional routes and has valued the highly developed skills and knowledge of expert practitioners as true clinical experts in their fields. Manley (2000a, 2000b) identifies the attributes, skills and processes required by consultant nurses, suggesting:

> 'If consultant nurses are appointed with the skills and processes described, they promise to be extremely influential in terms of the impact they will have on organisational culture and the subsequent positive effect on performance of individuals, teams and organisations.' (Manley 2000b p. 38).

Professional development for the expert or consultant nurse may not be in relation to career progression, but in terms of maintaining their expertise and being at the forefront of practice development. It will include sharing their expertise with others through writing and publishing and disseminating their work at conferences. It is likely to include debate and challenge with others operating at the same professional level, as well as developing skills of political leadership and influencing so that the voice of nursing is heard.

Summary

- Expert practitioners possess a unique and individualised knowledge and skill base that is embedded in their practice.
- They are at the top of their career level, and may become consultant nurses.
- Professional development needs are focused on expanding practice knowledge, creating and disseminating new knowledge and challenging others.

Activity

Part of professional development activity involves 'looking back–looking forward'. This exercise takes several minutes, so it is worth doing this when you have time to spare and can focus on it. It is also useful in terms of personal development planning, and therefore worth making notes as you go along.

Continued

Consider the features of practitioners at different stages in their development presented in Table 1.4.

Where are you now?
What makes you think that?
Where do you want to be?
Why?
What do you need to do to get there?
How will you do this?
When will you do it?
How long will it take?
How will you know you've got there?

A strategy for continuing professional development

Whilst it is useful to have a concept about what professional development of the individual practitioner may look like through the novice-to-expert continuum, most nurses will not be thinking in 'whole career' possibilities, but will take a much more pragmatic approach in terms of working out what they need to do next.

Models and frameworks tend to be academic structures, utilising concepts that have been developed for the model, and have particular and specific definitions. You will be introduced to many of these, relating to different aspects of professional development, throughout this book.

However, finding a way of guiding your own professional development, whether as a student or as a qualified nurse, need not be difficult or complicated. Nor does it need to be driven through a model or framework that requires you to understand the concepts involved before you can use it. The basic requirements for professional development are that it is:

- **R**elevant to your needs
- **E**asily defined
- **A**chievable in the time available (resources and other people)
- **C**ost effective
- **T**imely.

These key features, easily remembered as REACT, can be used to assess the practicality of any professional developmental activity that you may be considering. Various questions can be asked within these features that enable you to understand your motivation for the particular activity, and how you will go about planning to achieve it. This can direct your professional development activity, both by ensuring that whatever you choose to do is relevant for your work, and by structuring the processes that you will use to achieve it. In being very flexible (that is, you ask the questions) they can be applied to short, medium and long-term activity planning. I will be using this strategy, as will the other authors, throughout this book to show you how you can tailor it to where you are in your nursing career at the time, and how you can plan a range of activities to suit your needs.

The only words that you need to remember are:

- **W**hat?
- **W**hy?
- **W**hen?
- **W**here?
- **W**ho?
- **H**ow?

Collectively, these will be referred to as the 5WH cues. These are the question stems that you use to ask yourself:

- What kind of professional activity do you want to undertake?
- Why do you want to undertake it?
- When will you find the time to undertake it?
- Where will you undertake it?
- Who will support you?
- How will it be undertaken?

Relevant to your needs

Professional development activities that you undertake need to enable you to work better, and inform your practice as a nurse. This might seem obvious, but many practitioners have found that they start a programme of study only to find that they will not be able to use the new knowledge and skills or they are not appropriate or relevant for the work they are doing at the present time. Whilst you will undoubtedly learn from any activity that you do, if you do not use that learning in some way, it quickly becomes obsolete knowledge and forgotten; the new skills, if not practised, become rusty and may be dangerous and clumsy. It is important, therefore, to ask yourself a couple of questions when embarking on any professional development activity. These need to start with one of the trigger words. A couple of examples are:

- What areas of knowledge, skill or experience do I need to develop?
- Why do I want to develop these?
- How will this inform my practice?

Easily defined

This stage asks you to be specific in identifying your learning needs. This prevents you from taking directions which, although interesting, may have little relevance for what you really need to know. The key to defining the activity is to be able to identify the parameters that set its boundaries. Being able to phrase these with clarity, and being crystal clear about what you are trying to achieve may make the difference between success and failure. Defining your parameters gives you both a direction and a destination, and guides your activity. Questions you might ask are:

- What do I want to achieve?
- What underpinning knowledge do I need?
- What are my development objectives?
- What skills or competence do I need?
- How can I achieve these?

Achievable in the time you have available

Within a busy life we all need to fit work in alongside the demands of relationships and family, keeping house, leisure activities and other responsibilities and commitments. Professional development activity can be another drain on your time; the decision to start a degree course or a new specialist area of practice is a major undertaking. Even a short course or module of study will require you to learn new knowledge and skills, involve some process of assessment and require you to use your own time in addition to that freed from the workplace. The range of professional development activities shown in Figure 1.3 will involve different levels of commitment, time and resources. For instance, making time to search the library and access the electronic databases, to select relevant published papers, download and print them may be a challenge to fit in around your working day. First, you need to develop the basic information technology skills and an understanding of the library systems. Second, you need to be able to frame relevant search terms to ensure that you are effective in locating relevant literature. And, of course, that is just the start. Sometimes you will need to order offprints or source articles from inter-library loans. These may take weeks to come through the system. Once you have the materials to read, you then have to find the time to read them, analyse the content, synthesise the different perspectives being presented, evaluate the content, and draw conclusions about the relevance to your own practice. You may then want to record this activity in your professional portfolio.

In making the decision to engage in a professional development activity you need to make a commitment to seeing it through, otherwise not only are you wasting your time, but you also risk becoming disillusioned and losing confidence in your abilities to see something through. In order to do this, it is important to be honest with yourself and assess your own commitment and motivation so that you can plan to be successful and see it through to the end. It is far better to identify small activities that you know you will succeed at, than taking on large activities and not being able to complete them. Some questions that you may ask are:

- What time do I have available to commit to professional development?
- What types of professional development are achievable in this time?
- How can I re-order my life to achieve what I need to do?
- What resources can I draw on? For example access to libraries, funding, release from work.
- Who can I enlist to help me? For example colleagues, experts, academic staff, librarians, family, friends.
- Where can I find the physical space in which to study?

Cost-effective

All professional development comes at a cost, whether this be in hard cash terms, time spent away from the workplace or job role, or in a more esoteric way such as the cost of a nurse's own free time or self-funding activities. There is always a cash limited budget available within a workplace that will need to be applied for to fund activities, and applications for these monies will be assessed against the objectives for the work area and the needs for skills and knowledge. It may be that what is a priority for you is not a priority for your workplace when judged against other applications. This may result in you only being awarded part funding, or maybe none at all. Sometimes, you may need to decide whether you want to fund the activity yourself. Judgements need to be made for any staff development activity about whether the costs involved overall will result in sufficient benefit to the work area to warrant being spent.

Timely

This criterion is about doing the right activity at the right time in your life. Pre-registration students tend to start their programmes before they have family responsibilities because the commitment of time and energy needed for studying for a diploma or degree, over a three-year period is immense. Pre-registration programmes often require mobility around a geographical area, which can be more difficult if constrained by the need to take children to school, or a childminder, or to be there when they return home mid-afternoon. Hence, it is timely for intensive programmes to be studied when other life commitments are minimal. More mature students may enter pre-registration courses once children have gone to school or left home, or after caring for elderly relatives, for instance; again, when they have relatively more time for their studies. Honestly assessing the availability of appropriate amounts of time, often over long periods, will contribute to successful completion of your studies.

For qualified practitioners the pressure on time may be different. Being a professional practitioner involves a commitment to one's own development and this ultimately involves sacrificing some of your own time to do so. It is simply not possible to remain knowledgeable, and develop in your career only by using the time available to you at work. Engaging in formal study, such as studying for a degree, certainly requires the same sort of thought as when embarking on pre-registration courses. However, it is often 'fitted-in' to available time by making small adjustments to the way everyday life is organised. This often occurs when studying for a new qualification becomes important for career development or for progressing into new areas of practice. Questions you might ask yourself are:

- Why am I doing this now?
- What is the motivation for this activity in particular?
- What will be the result of this activity?

More informal types of professional development activities will arise and be stimulated by experiences and incidents in your practice. For instance, you may find yourself questioning whether you have sufficient knowledge to choose between alternative care strategies, or administer a drug that you have not met before and has been prescribed for a patient. Similarly, you may attend a training session and want more information. This is particularly important if you attend industry-sponsored activities such as drug company promotions, events organised by equipment manufacturers, or where free samples of products are available. Professional practitioners have a responsibility to ensure that their practice is evidence-based and that they are not unduly influenced by promotional considerations. This means that they need to consider alternatives to treatment and select the one most suited and appropriate for the person they are caring for. Being able to justify your decisions means you need to ensure you have sufficient knowledge and understanding to make informed decisions. This in itself may stimulate professional development activity.

Timely professional development means that whatever you learn will be immediately used in practice. This, in turn, reinforces the learning that has occurred and practice develops as a result. There is no space in most professionals' lives for the luxury of professional development activities that do not arise from and inform their practice. The link between professional development and professional practice is therefore indistinguishable.

Activity

It is worth putting this strategy into action while it is fresh in your mind.

Think back over your last shift. Is there anything that you can remember being unsure about and feeling that you needed to know more about?

Take this as a focus and ask yourself questions using the strategy.

Summary

- All professional development activity needs to be:
  — **R**elevant
  — **E**asily definable
  — **A**chievable
  — **C**ost effective
  — **T**imely
- A simple strategy for directing professional development activity is to ask yourself questions using the 5WH stems:
  — what?
  — why?
  — when?
  — where?
  — who?
  — how?

Chapter summary

This chapter has not only set the scene for this book, but has considered the context of professional development, a model through which professional nursing development can be understood in terms of knowledge and skills acquisition, and presented a strategy for considering professional development that will be refined and developed throughout the book. In so doing, it presents the differing faces of professional development, within which reflective practice and decision-making sit as essential components of professional practice today.

References

Benner, P. (1984) *From Novice to Expert: Excellence and Power.* Addison-Wesley, CA.

Department of Health (1999) *Making a Difference: Strengthening the Nursing, Midwifery and Health Visiting Contribution to Health and Health Care.* Her Majesty's Stationery Office (HMSO), London.

Department of Health (2000) *Continuous Professional Development: Quality in the NHS.* HMSO, London.

Department of Health (2001) *Working Together, Learning Together: a Framework for Lifelong Learning in the NHS*. HMSO, London.

Department of Health (2004) *Knowledge and Skills Framework*. HMSO, London.

Dreyfus, H.L. and Dreyfus, S.E. (1986) *Mind Over Matter*. Free Press, New York.

HSC 227 (1999) *Agenda for Change: Modernising the NHS Pay System*. Department of Health, London.

Jasper, M. (1999) Nurses' perception of the value of written reflection – the genesis of a grounded theory study. *Nurse Education Today*, **19**, 452–463.

Manley, K. (1997) A conceptual framework for advanced practice: an action research project operationalising an advanced practitioner/consultant nurse role. *Journal of Advanced Nursing*, **6** (3), 179–190.

Manley, K. (2000a) Organisational culture and consultant nurse outcomes: part 1, organisational culture. *Nursing Standard*, **14** (36), 34–38.

Manley, K. (2000b) Organisational culture and consultant nurse outcomes: part 2, nurse outcomes. *Nursing Standard*, **14** (37), 34–39.

National Committee of Inquiry into Higher Education (NCIHE) (1997) *Higher Education in the Learning Society; the Report of the National Committee of Inquiry into Higher Education (the Dearing Report)*. HMSO, Norwich.

Nursing and Midwifery Council (NMC) (2002) *An NMC Guide for Students of Nursing and Midwifery*. NMC, London.

Nursing and Midwifery Council (2004a) *The NMC Code of Professional Conduct: Standards for Conduct, Performance and Ethics*. NMC, London.

Nursing and Midwifery Council (2004b) *The PREP Handbook*. NMC, London.

Robinson, K., Eck, C., Keck, B. and Wells, N. (2003) The Vanderbilt Professional Nursing Practice Program: part 1: growing and supporting professional nursing practice. *Journal of Nursing Administration*, **33** (9), September, 441–450.

Spouse, J. (2003) *Professional Learning in Nursing*. Blackwell Publishing, Oxford.

Universities UK, SCOP, Universities Scotland, LTSN, QAA (2001) *Guidelines for HE Progress Files*.

Reflection and reflective practice

Learning objectives

Reflective practice is the way nurses learn from their experiences and develop their practice as a result. It is the main mechanism by which we develop as professionals throughout our working lives. This chapter explores the ways practitioners use the processes of reflection and reflective practice on the experiences they have within their working environment to learn and develop throughout their lives.

By the end of this chapter you will have:

- an understanding of the concepts of reflection and reflective practice
- an understanding of reflection as a learning strategy
- considered the benefits of practising reflectively
- explored the links between reflection and the generation of nursing and midwifery knowledge
- considered the value of knowledge arising from practice
- explored strategies for integrating reflection within professional practice and professional development.

The context of reflective practice

Take a couple of minutes to jot down some thoughts about these questions:

- How do professional practitioners continue to develop throughout their working lives?
- How does basic and initial knowledge and skill transform into expert knowledge and skill?
- How do we learn outside a formal learning environment?

It is hoped that these questions will already have got you thinking about the contents of this chapter. You know the beginnings of the answers to these questions because, as a successful human being, you have been learning every day of your life through the experiences you encounter. You also have experiences in clinical practice, whether as a student or as a qualified practitioner, that inform the way you practise and help you to identify the limits of your knowledge and skill.

This is the root of reflective learning and reflective practice. Very little of what we know comes from reading a book or sitting in a classroom setting. While we can be taught the basics, most of what we know comes from being successful in the things we do and learning to repeat this behaviour from an early age. Or, conversely, learning from our mistakes and trying not to repeat the behaviour. So, in a nutshell, reflective practice is about learning from our experiences and developing our practice as a result. Reflective learning is the process of learning from our experiences, reconsidering and rethinking our previous knowledge and adding this new learning to our knowledge base to inform our practice.

To be successful as professional practitioners, to develop and grow in that professional role, we need to be conscious of the ways we continually interact with our environment and build upon our knowledge base for practice. We need to be open to new challenges and to seek out new opportunities to continually develop our practice and, in consequence, develop as professional practitioners.

As students, we need to master different strategies for effective learning in the formal context: essay writing, taking notes, using computers and electronic databases, reading complex material – the list goes on. As student practitioners we also need to learn from clinical practice, by working with others, practising new skills, informing theory with practice and applying our knowledge to practice situations. Strategies for reflective learning straddle these two other learning scenarios, in that they help us to integrate the formal knowledge with the practical knowledge, and to learn by exploring everyday situations to help us make sense of and become comfortable and confident in an alien environment. Reflective learning skills do not stop on qualification; they develop further and become second nature to thinking professionals as they continue their own professional development throughout their careers. These skills are therefore considered to be *transferable* skills; you continue to draw on them and refer to them whenever you are in a working environment or need to adapt to something new.

This chapter introduces you to the basics of reflective practice and reflective learning strategies. It provides you with some practical skills which, like any other skill, need practice to become a part of the way you practise as a professional.

Setting the scene: reflection, reflective learning and reflective practice

Although notions of reflective practice have been around for a long time, the overt use of reflection as a learning strategy only became formally acknowledged in nursing education a couple of decades ago. This was linked with the recognition of reflective practice as the main way in which professionals learn in action (Schön 1983). As Chris Bulman (2004 p. 1) identifies:

> *'Nurses along with other professionals have been interested in and contributed to the growing body of literature on reflection because potentially it provides them with a vehicle through which they can communicate and justify the importance of practice and practice knowledge that derives from the realities of practice rather than purely from more traditional forms of knowing.'*

There are now many sound books and chapters outlining the theories of reflection, reflective practice and reflective learning (see further reading at the end of the chapter). It is sufficient here to reiterate the key concepts essential for understanding and using reflection as a strategy for learning and to inform practice.

First, and most fundamental, is Dewey's (1938) observation that 'we learn by doing and realising what came of what we did.' This refers to 'cause and effect': everything we do will have some sort of consequence, and the recognition that nothing happens in isolation; rather, that everything we do links to something that has happened to us, or we have done previously. A fundamental concept is the idea that we need to find ways of 'recognising' the causes and effects of our actions and acknowledging our own part in them. This makes the difference between practising consciously and unconsciously. A responsible and accountable practitioner clearly needs to be conscious of, and understand what they are doing. Conversely, the 'unconscious' practitioner (whilst not literally unconscious) follows routines and orders from others without questioning them and looking to develop and change their practice.

This leads us to the notions of what reflection is in itself and there is no universal definition above that of a dictionary definition. This draws attention to the idea of reflection as allowing us to 'see' ourselves in a physical sense, but also in a metaphorical sense to see 'within' ourselves. Reflection is also about seeing things again, and perhaps seeing them in a different way or from a different angle. The most concrete example of reflection is to look in a mirror. But, depending on the angle we look from, the curve of the mirror, or the distortion of the glass, we see a different picture. We also see it back to front, or the opposite of what other people see. At a more abstract level, we can take the idea of reflection as a way of looking at our practice from different angles, or perspectives.

The use of reflection in reflective practice and reflective learning, therefore, is about seeing inside or behind our experiences, seeing them from a different viewpoint, or with a different set of 'reflective lenses' in the spectacles through which we view our lives. So, a commonly used definition of reflective learning is that coined by Boyd and Fales (1983 p. 113):

> 'Reflective learning is the process of internally examining and exploring an issue of concern, triggered by an experience, which creates and clarifies meaning in terms of self and which results in a changed conceptual perspective.'

This is often coupled with the definition of Boud *et al.* (1985 p. 19):

> 'Reflection in the context of learning is a generic term for those intellectual and affective activities in which individuals engage to explore their experiences in order to lead to new understandings and appreciations.'

These are very academic definitions, and whilst they may be useful for those facilitating reflection, it is perhaps more relevant to consider a more recent definition that arises from working with health care professionals. For me, the concept of reflection that makes most sense, and is most accessible, comes from Gillie Bolton (2005), who presents the ides of 're-viewing' our experiences in multiple ways. She suggests that:

> 'Reflection is an in-depth consideration of events or situations outside of oneself: solitary, or with critical support. The reflector attempts to work out what happened, what they thought or felt about it, why, who was involved and when, and what these others might have experienced and thought and felt about it. It is looking at whole scenarios from as many angles as possible: people, relationships, situation, place, timing, chronol-

ogy, causality, connection, and so on, to make situations and people more comprehensible. This involves reviewing or reliving the experience to bring it into focus.' (Bolton 2005 p. 9)

In combination, these definitions tell us that reflective learning involves:

- learning from our experiences by reviewing them
- a thoughtful activity
- enabling us to understand something that has happened to us differently.

Reflective practice builds on the notions of reflection and reflective learning by adding some sort of action into the equation, thus:

Experience + reflection + learning → change in behaviour or action

This can be shown diagrammatically as the ERA cycle triangle. See Figure 2.1 (Jasper 2003 p. 2).

This makes it clear that reflective practice involves three basic components. First, there are the experiences that happen to us. These form the fundamental building block of reflective practice and give us the topics to reflect on. Hence, if we don't have experiences in practice we can't learn from them.

Second, we need to use reflective processes to work on these experiences to allow us to unlock the learning within them. There are many strategies and techniques for doing this, including models and frameworks that have been devised specifically for this purpose. But, this need not be complicated; it is more about getting into the habit of thinking over the things that have happened to you and trying to identify what you have learnt from them.

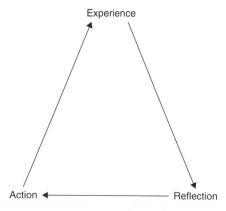

Figure 2.1 The ERA cycle. Reproduced with the permission of Nelson Thornes Ltd, from Jasper, M. (2003) *Beginning Reflective Practice.*

Finally, we need to contract with ourselves to take action as a result of the learning and understandings that have developed. Using reflection alone in order to learn is not reflective practice. Practice is about doing something; it is a *practical* activity. Therefore *reflective* practice means using the reflective processes to inform our practice in some way. It is one of the mental processes that enable us to transform our experiences into learning, and that learning into action. For a profession that is practice-based, and one that is learnt by developing that practice, the use of reflective learning is essential to maximise the learning opportunities that arise in the practice environment. For us to practise reflectively, we need to understand the processes that enable us to learn from experience, to develop a 'kitbag' of skills that will help us to do this, and to take a conscious decision to become 'reflective practitioners' in the way we conduct our practice. Therefore, reflective practice is all about taking action, and making some sort of change to our practice as a result of our reflective learning.

This concept is presented as a triangle because if one of the three parts is removed it no longer exists; this acts as a reminder that if reflection is not followed through to action then reflective practice isn't occurring.

Summary

- Reflection, reflective learning and reflective practice are all strategies to help us learn from our experiences in order to develop our understanding and inform our practice.
- Reflective learning involves actively thinking about our experiences in order to learn from them.
- Reflective practice involves three basic stages: experience, reflection and action.
- The final stage, taking action, is the key element of reflective practice.

Reflective practice as professional practice and development

Part of the responsibility of being a professional practitioner is to ensure that you give the best care possible to your patients and clients. In order to do that you need to continue to update your knowledge and skills base, and to build, in a continuous way, upon this basic knowledge as you gain experience, both as a student and as a practitioner. This learning never stops; the development of expertise is all about being open to new ideas, trying out new ways of doing things, and seeing possibilities for changes and developments to practice.

A reflective practitioner is constantly moving and changing their practice as they add in the learning gained from their experiences. Each time they come across something new, or which presents them with a challenge, they will subconsciously be scanning their memory banks to link it to something that has happened to them in the past. They then compare what they see in front of them with what they already know, and make decisions on the basis of this comparison. They may have to adapt previous strategies of what they know works and what may not, or need to get more information. They may decide to find some research-based evidence that will help them, or consult with others in order to come to a decision.

Benner (1984), in a landmark study of expertise in nursing, suggested that the expert practitioner 'operates from a deep understanding of the total situation', which many would refer to as 'professional intuition'. This is built up of a huge number of 'paradigm cases'[1] that act as the basis for an encyclopaedic professional knowledge carried around in their heads. This professional intuition has, in the past, been denigrated as unscientific, and therefore not to be trusted as dependable in a clinical context. However, if we rename intuition as 'professional expertise', built up and gained over years of experience, and tested in the clinical environment, it becomes a more robust concept (this is one of the debates at the heart of evidence-based practice and will be dealt with more fully in Chapter 5). After all, who would you rather see if you had a problem: a doctor with a couple of years' experience who has to look everything up in a book, and depends on population studies and clinical trials to predict the 'most likely' option, or an expert who can consider all of the available evidence, including that from his own experience, to devise an individualised treatment plan that relates specifically to you as a person?

'Intuitive' practice has been referred to as 'reflection in action' by Donald Schön (1983) who suggests that it is one of the ways professionals move beyond rule-bound behaviour to enable them to function in a world of uncertainty and see problems in a holistic way. It is the way that people think in action and theorise about practice while they are doing it. The features of reflection in action are:

- it is perceived as automatic
- it is seen as an unconscious activity
- it is often called 'intuitive' practice
- it results from a combination of knowledge, skills and practice
- it is difficult to articulate and explore.

This difficulty in articulation makes reflection in action difficult to explore and to use in any practical way. After all, if you ask someone to explain why they did what they did, they are likely to try to

[1] A paradigm case is a model, or reference case that sets a standard for us to refer to.

rationalise and provide theory to support their decisions, rather than being able to say what their thought processes were because these were subconscious. Rolfe *et al.* (2001) explore this concept further, tackling the intangible nature of reflection in action in a way that makes the concept easier to understand.

Activity

Reflection in action is a difficult concept to grasp without drawing on examples. One way is to think back over your last working day, and identify a particular patient you were working with. Make a list of the interaction you had with this patient, and where you were involved in making decisions about the care that could have had alternative actions.

If you were aware of consciously weighing up alternatives in your head, you were actively drawing on your knowledge and evidence base; this is one form of reflection in action. Then, what about those activities and decisions you took without 'thinking' about them? How did you know what to do? If you think about them more deeply, can you 'unpack' them in any way to uncover the knowledge and experiences that underpin your decision? We use reflection in action continually to inform what we do, and in making split-second decisions about our actions throughout our working day.

The other concept that Schön (1983) identified was 'reflection on action'. This is the conscious exploration of an event to discover more about it and learn from it. Reflection on action is:

- retrospective: it occurs after the event has happened
- a conscious, deliberative activity
- a cognitive process involving analysis, interpretation and recombination of information
- able to result in a new perspective being taken on the event
- an acknowledgement of the knowledge being used and results in knowledge deficits being identified
- an active process of transforming experience into knowledge
- able to contribute to the development of practice theory.

This makes it a more useful concept to work with, and is, in fact, at the basis of all deliberate reflective activity. As a concept it acknowledges the unique human experience bank that we have and uses this within an overt process of reflective exploration to unlock the understanding that we have of situations. This understanding is then used as the basis for our future actions in a cognitive way, that is it is the deliberate use of past experience to inform our practice. What may also emerge is that we have a knowledge deficit of some sort that we need to bridge, or we have some unresolved issues that have to be dealt with before we can feel comfortable with moving on.

Summary

- It is important for professional practitioners to continually update their knowledge and skills.
- Learning from clinical experiences is a valuable source of this updating.
- Reflection in action and reflection on action are the foundational processes used in reflective practice.
- Reflective practice, using reflection on action, is one of the main ways that professionals develop throughout their working lives.

The benefits of practising reflectively

Reflective practice is more than just a valuable learning tool for the practitioner. It also brings with it benefits for service users, your employers and your profession.

Activity

Take some time to think through the following questions. What are the benefits of reflective practice for:

- you?
- your patients and clients?
- your employer?
- your profession?

Benefits for the individual

My answers to the first of these – benefits for you as an individual practitioner – are in the list below. You may well have thought of a lot more. As an individual practitioner you will:

- ensure you are giving evidence-based care
- avoid routine practice
- focus on your patients as individuals rather than cases
- maximise your learning opportunities
- identify shortfalls in your knowledge and skills
- identify your learning needs
- value your own good practice
- continually develop your practice
- continually develop your own knowledge base
- create your own 'practice theory' (Rolfe *et al.* 2001).

These can be grouped together in three main ways:

- those that relate to the way you practise
- those that relate to your learning needs
- those that relate to the way you learn from your experiences in order to develop your practice.

These are the three cornerstones for professional development, in that they arise from your professional practice; they generate a continual stimulus for self-directed learning; and they help you to apply that learning to your practice. They can be represented as another triangle, demonstrating the interlinking of professional practice with continual learning. See Figure 2.2.

This ensures that your practice doesn't stand still, and that you are unlikely to sink into routine practice, or the all too common trap of doing things because 'that's the way we've always done it'. In terms of your own professional development, reflective practice and reflective learning ensure that you build upon your continually developing knowledge base arising out of your own interests as a professional practitioner. This means that nothing you do in order to develop is extraneous to providing care for your patients; it is this that drives your development.

How many times have you attended study days, or read articles, and thought 'That's interesting, I must remember to think about using that next time I come across something similar'? Or how often have you witnessed a different approach to care, given by someone else, and it has made you question the way you do things? And how many times have you actually followed these thoughts and ideas up, researched them a little further and then incorporated them into your caring practices?

Reflective practice provides a mechanism for doing this, for motivating you to follow through on those new ideas, on the articles you

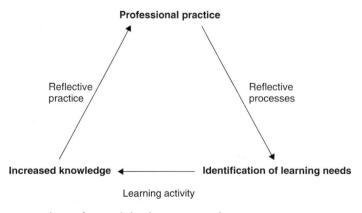

Figure 2.2 The professional development triangle.

read, and the presentations you go to, by providing the stimulus and strategies for turning information into action.

Benefits for patients and service users

As a result of your development and use of reflective practice, your patients will benefit by:

- receiving a better quality of care
- individualised and evidence-based care derived from their needs
- better standards of patient safety
- improved decision-making
- care using recent knowledge
- a reduction in the number of adverse patient incidents (such as drug errors, operating practice errors, falls)
- higher confidence in professional practitioners.

Benefits for patients arising from reflective practice tend to fall into the categories of quality and standards of care, and individualised care. Whilst evidence-based practice has brought with it the need to consider up-to-date research evidence and an awareness of the efficacy of treatment regimes, it can also mitigate against the unique needs of the individual patient. Reflective practice should prompt every nurse to consider each patient from an individual standpoint, with the patient being at the centre of their care, rather than the condition or illness that they are being treated for. Reflective practice helps us to see the patient as a whole, and consider all of their needs, ensuring that care packages are integrated rather than prescribed solely according to specific drug regimes. Consider Alan's story in Case study 2.1.

Alan's story demonstrates the importance of Jane's reflective practice for Alan's own particular set of circumstances. Alan, whilst suffering from diabetes, has a set of environmental and social circumstances which need to be considered alongside the research evidence and protocols that inform care of patients with that condition. Using the research evidence alone would not resolve Alan's problems; Jane's assessment and treatment plan, taking both the evidence and her experience and expertise into account, ensure that he has a treatment plan that is realistic for him, that he has played a part in devising and puts him and his needs at its centre. It is therefore more likely to be effective than if a rigid plan had been laid down that had not taken his unique circumstances into account. Jane's use of reflective practice and critical reflection, drawing from her own individualised knowledge base built up through experience, in combination with evidence-based knowledge, helped her to select from treatment options and, working in partnership with Alan, devise the most appropriate care package for his needs. She therefore gave both high quality care to Alan, and worked at the standards expected within the Diabetes NSF (DoH 2001),

---

Case study 2.1   Alan's story.

Alan has returned to Jane, a diabetic nurse consultant, for a six-month follow-up appointment. He was diagnosed as having diabetes a year ago and manages the condition, with the help of his wife, mainly through diet and carefully planning his daily schedules. At this appointment Jane notices that Alan looks run-down and listless, his skin has an unhealthy pallor, and he is limping, favouring his left foot. Jane follows a routine assessment process, to enable her to gather baseline data that she compares to his previous results, such as blood sugar levels, the balance of his diet, pulse recordings and his vision. However, despite these all being within normal ranges, Jane is concerned that Alan isn't in optimal health and explores further.

Alan has recently changed his working life and now works four thirteen-hour night shifts in the factory as a night-watchman as opposed to the daytime security work that he used to do. This has brought with it an increased salary, but he is finding that the long shifts are playing havoc with trying to eat at regular times and get a decent amount of sleep regularly. He fell over some boxes a couple of weeks ago and banged his left ankle, bruising it and breaking the skin. This hasn't healed as it would be expected to.

Jane draws on her understanding of diabetic complications, the NSF for diabetes and her previous experience of complications arising from living with diabetes. She also knows the importance of routine and diet for patients with diabetes and how they need to achieve a balance to maintain their health. Jane concludes that Alan's problems lie more with his lifestyle than with his physical condition. Together, they work out ways that Alan can manage his new job and work within the constraints imposed by his diabetes. Meanwhile, Jane considers the medical treatment needed for his ankle and ensures the relevant assessments are done and treatment regime started.

Alan is relieved that Jane has taken the time to consider him as a person, rather than just someone with diabetes, and leaves the consultation with a more positive attitude than when he arrived. He realises that he will be able to continue his new job, and that, with some help from his wife, he can control his diet and regain his previous levels of health.

---

by her employer, and by the Nursing and Midwifery Council within the *Code of Professional Conduct: Standards for Conduct, Performance and Ethics* (2004). In addition, she had the satisfaction of knowing that she had done the best she could for her patient, taking his unique circumstances into account and drawing on her own expertise and experience of caring for people with diabetes.

This sort of individualised care contributes to the quality of care received by service users and reduces the number of adverse patient incidents, or 'accidents' that can result when patients receive routine care, or protocols established that fail to treat the patient as an individual. This has knock-on implications for the employer, or organisation with which you work.

Benefits for your employer and the organisation you work for

Your employer or organisation will benefit from having reflective practitioners by achieving:

- a good reputation for professional practice
- higher standards and quality of care
- better recruitment and retention
- a multi-skilled workforce
- effective appraisal mechanisms, resulting in:
  - training and development needs arising from people awareness
  - reduced adverse patient 'incidents'
  - less litigation.

Care provider organisations are all regulated through inspection mechanisms and quality indicators designed to monitor standards across the health and social care sectors. The Health Care Commission was created to inspect NHS care providers according to specific criteria which apply to NHS providers nationally. These result in a 'star rating' being awarded to health trusts. In turn, this provides incentives for lower scoring trusts to work to improve their rating, whilst at the same time enabling the Government to identify 'failing' trusts that need stringent measures to help them improve the quality of their services. Trusts judged to be achieving high standards are further rewarded, with some now achieving 'foundation' status as flagship organisations within the NHS.

The use of reflective practice by all practitioners, in helping to raise the quality of care, also enables the employer to focus activity on specific targets by making these a measure of expectation for the practitioner. Certainly, trusts have to record patient complaints and adverse incidents in addition to standard measures such as waiting list times and bed-occupancy rates. Reflective practice enables practice development to tackle problem issues, resulting in better patient care, less adverse incidents and complaints, optimum use of available resources and the achievement of quality targets and standards.

Finally, I asked you to consider the benefits that might accrue for your profession as a result of reflective practice.

Benefits for your profession

The profession will benefit from:

- increased public confidence
- increased inter-professional parity

- raised professional profile and standing
- developing the nursing knowledge base
- recognition of nursing specific skills
- recognition of the unique contribution that nursing makes to patient care.

Nursing and midwifery are regulated, by law, by a professional body charged with 'protecting the public through professional standards' (NMC 2004). It is the Nursing and Midwifery Council's role to ensure that anyone practising as a registered nurse, midwife or specialist community public health nurse meets minimum specified standards within their practice. However, the NMC, together with the professional organisations, such as the Royal Colleges of Nursing and Midwives, and the Community Practitioners and Health Visitors Association, are also charged with representing the professions at Governmental level, and promoting the role of nurses as professional practitioners. As a result, they also have a role in ensuring the continuing education and consequent status development of nurses.

The last two decades have witnessed the improving status of nurses, midwives and specialist community public health nurses as a result not only of large scale changes to the national health service in Britain, but also in recognition of the increasing technicality and specialisation of nursing roles, demanding individualised expertise and continual professional development. This, to some extent, is what prompted the NMC PREP standards (formerly devised by the UKCC) as a way of ensuring the development of competent independent practice, and that the roles, such as specialist and consultant nurses, conform to specified standards. Whilst the debate still continues in terms of what is meant by advanced practice and how this can be measured, it is the intention of the NMC to introduce the higher level of the nursing register soon, bringing with it recognition of those practitioners who are visibly practising as experts in their own right.

Having all registered practitioners practising as reflective practitioners therefore brings with it ways of developing and promoting the status and dependability of the professions themselves. We are increasingly seeing significance of the role of nursing being promoted as contributing to developments in patient health. For instance, Professor Christine Beesley was made responsible for improving hygiene in hospitals and reducing hospital acquired infections such as methicillin resistant *Staphylococcus aureus* (MRSA) when she took over the Chief Nursing Officer's role at the Department of Health in 2004.

In addition, reflective practice enables 'practice theory' (Rolfe *et al.* 2001) to be recognised and disseminated, as more nurses become overtly aware of the knowledge behind their everyday practice. The past three decades have seen a huge increase in the number of books and journals that track the development of nursing theory in its own right, as opposed to an adjunct of medicine, psychology, pharmacology or any other of the specific knowledge bases that contribute to understanding patient care. Nurse education moved into higher education in Britain in the late 1980s; thus, we now have more than a decade of nurses educated to diploma level as a minimum, with many more having studied degrees in nursing at Bachelor's and Master's levels. There are professors of nursing standing alongside professors of other disciplines, bearing witness to the development of nursing as an academic, as well as a practice discipline.

Reflective practitioners function as independent professionals at all levels of their practice. This therefore contributes to the developing status of the profession in both the public's eyes, and those of the other professions, bringing with it a recognition of the unique contribution that skilled nurses and midwives make to patient care.

Summary

Practising reflectively results in benefits for:

- the individual, in terms of providing individualised care, identifying their learning needs, and learning from experience
- the patient, in terms of higher quality and standards of care, and care designed to meet their own unique needs
- the employer, in terms of standards of care achieved, in having a continuingly developing workforce which recognises its own professional development needs
- the profession, in terms of self-regulation of the practitioners, in developing nursing's knowledge base, in contributing to increasing the status of nursing and recognition of nurses' contribution to patient care.

Tools for reflective practice

Becoming a reflective practitioner involves conscious decision-making. It is a deliberative approach which requires activity and effort on the part of the person doing it. Whilst we can, and do, reflect in an unconscious way, and gradually build up a repertoire of skills as a result, in order to make the most of our experiences and learning in an active way we need to embrace the notion of reflection as a learning tool and build up our skills by practicing in the same way as we learn any other skill. Reflection may come naturally to some of us; to others it will present more of a challenge, but everyone can learn to be a reflective practitioner if they have the commitment to do so, and take the opportunities that arise during their lives to form the basis for that reflection.

The ERA (experience–reflection–action) triangle provides a guide for directing our reflective practice, by drawing attention to the work that needs to be done at each stage.

Experience, choosing a focus for reflection, the first side of the triangle

Common sense tells us that we cannot stop our everyday activities in order to take time out to reflect on everything that happens to us. First of all, we wouldn't get anything else done. Second, as with any activity, we need variety otherwise we become stale and bored; the activity ceases to be effective. We need, instead, to use reflection as a focused activity within a particular timeframe in order to make the most of it and as one of the strategies we use in our working lives as practitioners.

So, in choosing a focus for reflection we need to have some sort of guide, or parameters, that help us to select key experiences we can learn from. The four criteria below, using the acronym SODA, help to select experiences for reflective activity.

(1) **Significance:** the experience must stand out in some way.
    (a) It might be the first time you have encountered it.
    (b) It is unusual in some way.
    (c) It is memorable in some way; it stands out in your mind.
    (d) It may bring out an emotional response in you: happy, sad, angry, or proud.
    (e) It may relate to a specific learning outcome you want to achieve such as demonstrating a practice skill, completing an academic assignment, developing your knowledge.
(2) **Outcome:** it needs to provide a developmental opportunity for you, such as:
    (a) an increased understanding of a situation
    (b) identifying a knowledge deficit or learning need
    (c) resulting in a new knowledge or skill within your practice
    (d) developing an insight into your own behaviour or thought processes
    (e) taking a different perspective on an experience.
(3) **Describable:** it must be sufficiently complete in itself for you to be able to describe it:
    (a) It needs to have identifiable boundaries, such as a timeframe; a patient experience or encounter; an encounter with another person; an event that happens; something that you have witnessed; etc.
    (b) You must be able to remember sufficient detail to give a complete picture to another person (even if no one else ever sees it).

(c) You need to be aware of the consequences, for yourself and for others involved, in using incidents in a public way; they may have implications for them, or for you.

(e) Be aware of issues of confidentiality.

(4) **Action:** it needs to result in some action being taken, such as:

(a) finding out more information

(b) developing a new skill

(c) changing your and/or others' practice

(d) talking the situation over with another person

(e) seeking further help.

Using these criteria, you can choose any experience you have, as long as you are choosing it for a particular reason and it will satisfy some particular need that you have. Whilst most of the time you will select experiences that happen to you in a work situation, sometimes you might want to learn to recognise your own skills and characteristics. For instance, you can learn a great deal about how you react in emergency situations by reflecting on how you coped with a home disaster such as the central heating failing, or a power cut that occurred when you were away on holiday.

Activity

Identify an out-of-the-ordinary situation from your past personal or professional life that you dealt with successfully. Use questions arising from SODA and the 5WH cues to explore the incident. Some examples are:

S Why was it significant?
Why does it stand out in your mind?
What is important about this incident?

O What did you want to achieve as a result of dealing with it?
What might you learn from it to help your practice?
What might you learn about yourself?

D How can you describe it?
What are the parameters of the incident?
What may be the consequences, for you and others, of exploring the incident?
What ethical issues must you consider, for example confidentiality?
What are the professional implications of exploring the incident?

A What action might need to be taken?
Who else can help you?

Having selected an experience to reflect on, with a particular purpose in mind, you can now explore these in more detail using the reflective processes.

Summary

- The ERA triangle can be used to direct your reflective activity.
- Any experience that you have can form the basis for reflective activity.
- The experiences need to be chosen for their significance, outcome, describability, and action.

Using the reflective processes, the second side of the triangle

If you completed the activity above you will already have started using the reflective processes that enable us to think more deeply about our experiences and learn from them.

Using frameworks and models

Fundamentally, being reflective means being willing to ask questions about something. The secret, skill and risk, is to find the most appropriate questions to ask that will lead you to the outcome you want to achieve. With a bit of practice, you will know the questions to ask, but most 'beginning' reflectors start off using a framework or model of reflection that will guide them through the process. Very often, students will be introduced to one or two frameworks through the course they are studying, and may be required to use these for their reflective activity. However, there are many frameworks available, and each will have been developed from a particular starting point, depending on why it was created in the first place. The frameworks lead the reflector in a particular direction. This may be:

- identifying the knowledge that was being used in an activity
- identifying learning from an experience
- recognising individual development
- developing practice
- learning about ourselves
- to demonstrate our accountability as professional practitioners.

Frameworks characteristically arise from their creator's value base, be this from an educational basis (for example Gibbs 1988) from a practice basis (for example Johns 1998) or from a personal/professional developmental basis (Borton 1970; Rolfe *et al.* 2001; Bolton 2005). The frameworks often consist of cue questions, based on and focused through fundamental key concepts. The framework provides a checklist for the practitioner to work through, answering and considering the cue questions as they progress. Fundamentally, they draw on the concepts of experiential learning identified as:

- people learn best from their own experiences
- what people do is more important than what they know

- rendering behaviours and attitudes visible enables them to be explored and addressed
- people need to come to their own understanding, rather than be told how to think or behave
- moving beyond knowledge and into skill by generating a learning experience
- achieving change in behaviour and attitude
- the learning process, to be effective, needs to be enjoyable, motivating and rewarding. (www.teamskillstraining.co.uk).

The frameworks also develop the 'experiential learning cycle' consisting of four stages proposed by Kolb (1984):

- concrete experience
- reflective observation
- abstract conceptualisation
- active experimentation.

These are further related by Kolb to the predominant *learning style* that we all have, recognising that we all have preferred ways of learning that enable us to be more effective in the way we assimilate new knowledge into the way we behave and practise.

Pre-established frameworks have a number of advantages:

- They have been designed for a particular purpose, and tested and therefore can provide a predictable end result.
- They enable the reflector to work through a predetermined set of questions.
- They direct the reflective activity, enabling the reflector to focus on the outcomes of the activity rather than the processes themselves.
- They are independent of the reflector, and although they can be manipulated, tend to be used in their entirety.
- They challenge the reflector by (often) going in directions, and asking questions that the reflector would not ask themselves.
- They result in a new perspective being taken on the experience.
- They can be used in a variety of different ways:
  — to guide individual reflection
  — used verbally, within a supervisory relationship
  — informally reflecting with others, or within group discussions and activities
  — to guide written reflection.

However, they can also restrict reflective activity by:

- directing the reflector in a specific direction
- directing the nature of the outcome
- requiring understanding of the nature of the concepts within them
- limiting the reflector's own imagination and creativity
- fixing the reflector within one framework

- limiting flexibility to the cue questions being asked
- being used inappropriately.

Frameworks and models certainly have a place in stimulating and guiding reflective activity, and are extremely useful tools for anyone wanting to try out approaches different to their everyday thought processes. However, the rider to this is that it is important to select a framework that helps you to achieve what you want from your reflective activity, not that confines you and dictates where that activity goes. Indeed, Chris Johns (2004 p. 19) suggests that 'the risk is that practitioners will fit their experience to the model of reflection rather than use the model creatively to guide them to see self within the context of the particular experience'. Gillie Bolton takes this point even further when she says:

> 'Giving students set pro formas, lists of prompts, questions or areas which must be covered in reflective practice will stultify, make for passivity and lack of respect. Professionals need to ask and attempt to answer their own questions.' (Bolton 2005 p. 82)

These views aside, however, many educators believe that students benefit, at least initially, from learning to reflect through a particular framework or perspective. Students also often find that a framework enables them to concentrate on developing reflective skills without having to worry about the process of doing it, and appreciate having a strategy for reflection offered. However, at the end of the day this is about personal choice, and I have certainly found that once students and practitioners have mastered the basic skills, they like to move from given frameworks to strategies that allow them to ask and answer their questions in a way that works for them.

Key to making a choice about using a framework is having an understanding of the differences between the published frameworks and models. It is also vital that the principles behind the framework, and the course being studied, or the practitioner's own world view is consonant. An analysis and comparison between some of the common frameworks, and others that have been published is presented in Table 2.1.

In selecting a pre-formatted framework, it is worth working through the set of questions in Box 2.1 to ensure you choose the one most appropriate and likely to help you achieve your aims.

Summary

- Frameworks and models for reflection provide useful guidance for reflective activity.
- They are particularly useful for the novice reflector, those wanting to find a different perspective, or those wanting to challenge the way they habitually think.

- All frameworks are devised from a specific perspective, and designed to guide the reflector in a particular way.
- Frameworks need to be selected as appropriate for the purpose the reflector wants to achieve and coherent with the practitioner's own values underpinning their practice.

Creating a framework for reflection

Once the principles of reflection, reflective learning and reflective practice have been absorbed and internalised, and the skills for reflection developed, the practitioner will have created a knowledge and skills base to be able to reflect flexibly, selecting from available frameworks if necessary, or creating their own to suit their needs.

The majority of published frameworks and models include six stages (Jasper 2003):

Stage one: selecting a critical incident to reflect on
Stage two: observing and describing the experience
Stage three: analysing the experience
Stage four: interpreting the experience
Stage five: exploring alternatives
Stage six: framing action

Indeed, these summarise the reflective processes that any reflective activity encompasses. These can form the basis for creating your own framework for reflection according to the purpose you want to use it for. They simply summarise the processes involved in the reflective cycle, as opposed to presenting specific cue questions or directions and outcomes for the reflector to achieve. If the personal aspects specific to each practitioner are incorporated within each stage, this becomes a working framework for helping a practitioner to ask the questions about their practice without a superimposed agenda. The questions can be directed by using the 5WH cues. Case study 2.2 illustrates how this can work.

This case study illustrates the selective nature of using a framework to achieve the end that you want. Clearly, this student wanted to resolve several issues in her own mind and worked through questions that would enable her to do this. The final question asks her what her perspective on the situation is now she has worked through a reflective process. This enables the practitioner to identify any lingering issues and tackle them through another reflective cycle.

Using this flexible approach, rather than a directive framework, enables the practitioner to direct her energies to where the most important issues are, rather than being drawn down lines of questioning that would not necessarily help her to work on the situation as she needs to.

Table 2.1 A comparison of published frameworks for reflection.

Author/s	Title of the framework	Perspective	Presentation	Key cues/questions
Borton (1970)		Developmental	Three developmental questions Linear	Question stems of: what? so what? and now what? Asks the reflector to create the rest of the question
Mezirow (1981)	*Levels of Reflectivity*	Learning	Two main levels, each subdivided into three subsections	Consciousness level, affective reflectivity, discriminating, judgemental Critical consciousness level, conceptual, psychic, theoretical
Boyd and Fales (1983)	*Stages of Reflection*	Individual learning	Six stages Linear	A sense of inner discomfort Identification or clarification of concern Openness to new information from external and internal sources Resolution Establishing continuity of self with past, present and future Deciding whether to act on the outcome of the reflective process
Kolb (1984)	*Kolb's Experiential Learning Cycle*	Individual learning	Cycle of four stages	Concrete experience, reflective observation, abstract conceptualisation, active experimentation
Goodman (1984)	*Levels of Reflection*	Individual learning	Three levels – linear	1st level – reflection to reach given objectives 2nd level – reflection on the relationship between principles and practice 3rd level – reflection which besides the above incorporates ethical and political concerns
Gibbs (1988)	*Gibbs' Reflective Cycle*	Individual learning	Cycle of six stages	Description: what happened? Feelings: what were you thinking and feeling? Evaluation: what was good and bad? Analysis: what sense can you make of the situation? Conclusion: what else could you have done? Action plan: if it arose again what would you do?

Holm and Stephenson (1994)	*A Practitioner's Framework for Reflection*	Individual practice development	List of cue questions – linear	Choose a situation – ask yourself nine questions, for example: What was my role in this situation? What actions did I take? How could I have improved the situation?
Kim (1999)	*Critical Reflective Inquiry*	Reflective research	Three levels in increasing complexity – linear	Descriptive level of reflection; Theory and knowledge building level of reflection; Action-oriented level of reflection
Rolfe, Freshwater and Jasper (2001)	*A Framework for Reflexive Practice*	Practice development	Combines several theorists concepts into a developmental framework	Uses Kim's (1999) three levels of reflection, structured through Borton's three cue questions, incorporated into Gibb's cycle and supplemented by John's cue questions
Bolton (2001–2005)	*Through the Looking Glass*[1]	Learning	Narrative writing with critical reflection and group discussion	Writing stories about a closely observed event; Critical reflection on the event; Critical discussion; Event re-explored through further writing
Johns (1991–2004)	*Model for Structured Reflection*	Understanding and learning, developmental	Continually developed since 1991. The 2004 version is fourteenth. Although structured through a series of questions, author emphasises the dynamic nature of the model	Version 14 comprises 16 cues which incorporate Carper's (1978) four ways of knowing: aesthetics, empirics, personal, ethics plus reflexivity. Examples of cues are: Bring the mind home; What was I trying to achieve and did I respond effectively? How does this situation connect with previous experiences? What would be the consequences of alternative actions for the patient, others and me?

[1] I have taken the liberty of extracting the features of this approach from Gillie Bolton's (2005) book – she herself does not present this as a model nor claim it to be so. Hence, if I have misrepresented this, the error is mine alone.

Box 2.1 Criteria for selecting a reflective framework.

What am I trying to achieve?

- my own learning or identification of my learning needs
- increased understanding
- to take a different perspective on an experience or event
- practice development.

How do I want to reflect?

- in my head
- verbally – in a dialogue, in a group, with facilitation
- in writing.

Who do I want to reflect with?

- myself
- one other person
- other colleagues/students
- my supervisor/academic tutor
- another group of people.

What sort of structure do I want to use?

- broad questions
- specific questions
- a reflective cycle
- a framework that leads me towards action
- a framework that leads me towards a deeper understanding
- a facilitative and developmental framework.

When do I want to reflect?

- immediately
- after I get home from work
- during the next session in university
- during clinical supervision
- at some other convenient time.

Where do I want to reflect?

- within the clinical environment
- at home
- at university
- in a quiet area away from the clinical environment
- in a neutral place.

What are the values underpinning and inherent to the model?
   How do these fit with my own values as a practitioner?

Case study 2.2   Juggling time.

It was my last week on Peace Ward, a 32-bedded rehabilitation unit for young people recovering from brain injuries. The patients have complex needs encompassing not only physical recovery from road traffic accidents or cerebrovascular accidents, but they are also coming to terms with psychological and emotional challenges such as changing body image, potential lifestyle changes, potential dependency and changes to their skills for employment. They may also have to deal with long-term paralysis and the consequences of that for their sexuality and relationships.

What stands out in your mind as significant during that week? (stage one)
Many things happened, but there is one I found very upsetting. Joe, aged 40, had had a stroke four months ago. Initially, he found it difficult to accept this had happened to him, and he rejected accessing services or rehabilitation as a way of denying the reality of his situation. Instead, he tried continuing his work from his home computer and did not address his immediate needs consequent from the stroke. By the time the bleeding in his brain had stopped and he accepted he needed help he was suffering from a left-sided hemiplegia. His speech was unaffected, but he was extremely emotionally volatile and had become quite paranoid about the motives of everyone who was trying to help him. This led us to believe that he was cognitively impaired as a result of the stroke, making it difficult for him to accept treatment and options for both the short and medium term. He had resisted both physiotherapy and occupational therapy when he judged they were not appropriate, making it difficult for the therapists to work on an agreed plan of therapy. He was also a heavy smoker and had a poor diet, despite being an educated professional. His smoking behaviour made it difficult for him to accept in-patient care in the unit, as his smoking was necessarily restricted. It was this that led to the incident below.

What happened?
I was responsible (supervised by the ward manager) for a group of six patients, including Joe, that day. Joe was returning from his morning physiotherapy, walking alongside Kerry, dragging his left leg. He refuses to use a walking aid such as a stick, or to be supported by others. He wanted a cigarette and wanted Kerry to go outside with him while he smoked. Kerry refused, saying that she was too busy, but also that she didn't want to breathe in the smoke or come into contact with it in any way. She said she would take him outside but then leave him by himself in a safe place, and return for him in ten minutes. Joe immediately became very angry and started shouting at Kerry. I was in the office at the top of the ward at the time and heard raised voices and went to explore. I saw Joe raise his hand as if to strike Kerry, and called to him to stop. In doing so he overbalanced, fell and hit his head on the wall. I called for help and tried to assess Joe's physical situation. He was not unconscious but was

Continued

struggling to get up. He pushed me away and tried to hit me. He was shouting at me to leave him alone and trying to push me away. He hit me in the ribs and I fell onto the floor too, hurting my back when I landed. More people arrived, and the ward manager took over, directing getting Joe into a chair and back to bed, calling the house officer and telling me to complete the accident report. She completely cut me out of the caring process, leaving me to follow on and do what I was told, even though Joe was part of my group of patients and I had worked with him for over three months during his rehabilitation.

How did this make you feel? (stage two)
I have mixed feelings.

First of all, I was shocked that Joe had been so violent and that I was potentially in danger. I was shaking, my ribs hurt and my back was jarred, causing me problems. I couldn't understand why he was trying to hurt me when all I was doing was trying to help him.

Second, I was worried about Kerry and the effect this would have on her. She clearly felt responsible for 'winding Joe up' and the fact that he had become angry and violent. I wanted to talk to her about what had happened.

Third, I am worried that I did something wrong and that the ward manager sees me as incompetent because of the way I dealt with the situation. She took over completely and hasn't spoken to me about it at all. In fact she seems to be quite angry with me. I don't understand why.

Finally, I am worried that I might have caused Joe to be hurt further because I called out to him to stop. He now has a bruised face on his left side and is having visual problems.

What were you trying to do? (stage three)
Initially, I wanted to stop Joe hitting Kerry so I told him to stop. After he fell, I was trying to assess any damage and his condition, and ensure his safety. I didn't notice my ribs and back until later. When the ward manager took charge, I just did as I was told.

Why did you act as you did? (stage four)
Well, I have a duty of care to my patients and those I work with. I couldn't just watch Joe strike Kerry so I had to intervene. When he fell I needed to ensure he wasn't in immediate danger. I needed to get help as it wouldn't be safe to get him to his feet and try to walk him into the ward. He was also potentially violent and was refusing help; he just kept shouting and was angry. He accused Kerry and me of making him fall and it all being our fault. I realise that he is emotionally unstable, and that this sort of violent behaviour is often a result of having a stroke. It is just so hard to remember this is likely to happen, as most of the time Joe is so rational and acts like a gentleman.

I think I was probably shocked and went into automatic behaviour when the ward manager took over. Initially, I was grateful that someone else was in charge, and relieved that I didn't have to make the decisions. But now I am cross that she didn't facilitate me to make the decisions and handle the situation completely. After all, I am nearly qualified now and need to have this experience. I would have preferred her to ask me what I would do and allow me to get on with it, rather than just taking over.

What could you have done differently? (stage five)

(1) *The trigger to the incident.* I knew Joe would want a smoke on return from physiotherapy, and I knew Kerry would not want to accompany him. In future I would anticipate this and make arrangements prior to his return, so that he knew in advance he'd be able to have his cigarette. It is difficult for him to work to a regime, but I think we could compromise and meet halfway about when and where he smokes. I also feel that we have a role as health promoters and health educators, and that we need to reinforce the threats to his health of continuing to smoke. This needs to be part of his recovery package and perhaps he needs some cognitive therapy to enable him to tackle his smoking.

(2) *Shouting at Joe.* This was an automatic reaction to what I saw happening. I don't think I would do anything differently if this happened again. I was trying to protect Kerry, and this worked effectively.

(3) *Handling the fall.* Again, I would call for help and assess the situation. I did, however, put myself in danger. How could I avoid that? Looking back, I probably did not talk to Joe before I touched him and maybe he thought I was trying to do something to him. I need to remember that people get frightened in situations like this and can react violently. I need to remember to protect myself.

(4) *The ward manager taking over.* I do understand that she was responsible overall for the care of the patient and for me as a member of staff. I know that she was trying to manage the whole situation for everyone's benefit and that she was not deliberately undermining me. In fact, she may not be aware of how I felt. I would not have been her first priority at all. Perhaps I could have been more assertive, rather than just letting her get on with it. I could have made suggestions to show that I know what to do, such as offering to call the house officer and filling in the accident form. So, I think it is up to me to talk to her about what happened and how I felt.

What are you going to do now? (stage six)

Talk to the ward manager and use this as a learning experience in managing incidents – something like this doesn't happen every day and I need to make the most of the experience. I also need to reassure the ward manager that I am not useless in emergencies and that I did know what to do.

I need to talk it over with Kerry and help her reflect on the incident.

I need to talk to Joe about what happened and make sure he doesn't think I blame him in any way.

I need to think more carefully before approaching a potentially violent situation and work out the risks before I engage.

Continued

I need to think forward when planning care for patients and work with their individual needs in a partnership; this whole incident could probably have been avoided.

I need to read up on the emotional and cognitive effects of strokes. I wonder whether Joe would accept help from a psychologist in terms of managing his anger and emotions. Perhaps I'll talk to one of them and see if it would be an appropriate referral.

How do you feel now?
I understand that these sorts of things will always happen and that my role is to manage them with the least damage to anyone. Although I was hurt by the ward manager's actions I do now understand why she acted as she did. I have identified my learning needs, and how I might do things differently in another situation. I also understand my own coping processes better. I have learnt a lot from reflecting on the incident and now no longer feel guilty or upset about what happened.

Summary

- The reflective processes can be six basic stages.
- These can be used to direct reflective activity as appropriate for the practitioner.
- This enables reflection to be focused on the issues significant to the individual.

Putting the 'action' into reflective practice, the third side of the triangle

A great deal of work, time and energy goes into the reflective processes. It usually results in seeing things differently as a result of the 'reviewing' process and provides a new perspective on the event or incident. This may be enough for you. Certainly, taking a different perspective on something that has been causing you to use your mental energy, by worrying or fretting, by being angry or resentful, will be some sort of resolution in itself because it helps you to move on from the event. However, you will also have generated a lot of energy; anything that helps you to turn a negative or uncomfortable awareness into one that is positive changes the way you see it and motivates you into doing something. This section is about following through on that energy and contracting with yourself to turn learning into action.

Most practitioners are practical people; they like doing something as a result of assessing a situation and working out a course of action. It follows, therefore, that some sort of action should result from reflective activity. What a waste of time it would be if you saw a patient for the first time, ran a battery of diagnostic tests, used your experience to ask them the right questions to come up with a diagnosis about their problems, formulated a plan of action to help them resolve them, and then did nothing.

Healer, heal thyself.

Reflective practice is the personal tool of the practitioner; it is primarily for you and your own learning practice and life. Learning changes practice; professional development will not happen unless you complete the ERA triangle and turn the understanding and learning from your reflective activity into action.

What sort of action?

If you have worked your way through the reflective processes, either using a framework or devising your own strategy, you will have ended up with a plan of action. This arises as a logical deductive process from your introspection of your experiences. The previous case study illustrates how this happens; it just needs the student to push herself into doing the things she has diagnosed for herself. Of course, some will be a lot easier than others. Some will be more immediate than others; some will be short term; others can be delayed; whilst others relate to the way practice is carried out in the long term and may involve wholesale changes to values and conduct.

In the same way that being reflective is a deliberate decision, so is taking action to complete the ERA cycle; being reflective alone is not sufficient to be a reflective practitioner. A reflective practitioner is not a person who sits around having reflective thoughts all day. A reflective practitioner is one who changes things as a result, who gets up and informs their practice with the result of their reflective activity. A reflective practitioner makes things happen.

Summary

- Action needs to happen as a result of the reflective processes.
- Action is another deliberative decision made as part of the ERA cycle.
- Reflective practice does not occur without action being taken.

Micro-methods for reflective practice

In this section I will suggest some methods for reflecting, the 'how' of reflective practice that helps to make sense of the reflective processes and frameworks or models if you choose to use them. In Box 2.1 I suggested some criteria that you may wish to use when selecting a framework for reflection. You were asked to consider how you want to reflect and who you want to reflect with.

How you reflect, using micro-strategies

There is one main decision to be made here: are you going to reflect only in your head, will you be reflecting with others, or will you be writing as part of your reflective activity? Reflective writing has the next chapter to itself, and links with Chapter 6 on portfolios and evidence, too. Here, I want to concentrate on cognitive reflection as a process that is a thinking or verbal activity.

Reflection as a way of practice needs to be relatively simple to do, quick, have immediate outcomes, result in an action plan and be flexible for use. One way of doing this is to carry around with you a mental framework for reflection on action. Gibbs' (1988) framework, consisting of six stages, is useful for this (see Table 2.1).

Using the 5WH cues

However, a simpler framework arises from the 5WH question stems I introduced in Chapter 1, using:

- what?
- why?
- when?
- where?
- who?
- how?

These are very easy to remember and have the advantage of enabling you to focus the question on the particular event or outcome you want to achieve. In this chapter I want to focus on using the cues to select an experience to reflect upon. In Chapter 3, these are expanded into a framework for reflection that can be used through the reflective processes themselves. Basically, you use these to ask yourself questions, ensuring that you complete the ERA cycle. Some examples of questions using these stems are shown in Table 2.2.

'What' questions

'What' questions help you to set the parameters for your reflections. This may seem to be a formal and over-complicated start to the process, and of course it is not absolutely necessary. In fact, Bolton (2005) suggests that the way to start reflective writing is to simply make yourself spend a few minutes (giving yourself a time limit) writing about whatever comes into your head. She believes that significant issues will come to the fore and enable you to write. But, for many people this approach may lack focus, especially if there are certain issues that you know you want to write about. It also does not really apply to mental reflection, or in having reflective conversations with others, which always start with some sort of trigger or cue. The majority of theorists

Table 2.2 Examples of questions using the 5WH cues.

What	Why
do you want to write about? is the purpose of reflecting on this? do I want to learn/achieve? may be the outcome?	am I reflecting on this? is this important?
When	**Where**
can I explore it more thoroughly? do I need to resolve it? do I need to take action?	can I find the space to reflect on it further? is the equipment I need to write, for example computer, desk, Internet access? am I most comfortable writing?
Who	**How**
may be affected if I reflect on this experience? else do I need to involve (if anyone)?	can I reflect on this incident most effectively? can I learn from this?

who have created reflective frameworks suggest that the start to the reflective process is to deliberatively select an experience to reflect on. Asking 'what' questions helps you to identify, from all of the experiences you have, those that require further and extensive exploration. This purposeful selection helps to avoid spending time on less significant events, and to some extent, helps you not to avoid those big issues that need dealing with, or are stopping you from moving on in some way. Some key questions are:

- What do you want to reflect on? This might be a critical incident at work, a patient episode, a training event or study day, something you have read, something you need to read about, a knowledge deficit, something that has caused you to respond in an emotional way, something that is unresolved. The key criterion is that it is something that will result in learning, that will inform the care you provide to patients, and will contribute to your professional development.
- What is the purpose of reflecting on it? Consider the outcome you want, such as resolving an issue or arriving at a solution, increasing your knowledge and understanding, developing a skill, completing an assignment or assessed piece of work, identifying your learning. Ensuring you are clear about your outcomes helps you to focus on the essential components of the reflection and keeps you on track.
- What will you do with it? It may be that working with an experience using reflection ends with a mental or emotional resolution to

it, and you need take no further action. However, reflection may help in clarifying professional issues and ascertaining courses of action, but then need action to be taken. Anticipating what the potential or possible outcomes may be, before you start exploring an issue, may help you to select the strategy for exploring them, or perhaps protect or warn you about consequences that may have further repercussions. For instance, it may be that you need to take an issue to a higher authority, or to tackle another person's practice. There may be issues of professional misconduct or criminal negligence that will clearly involve others. An illustration of this is the decision to use the whistle-blowing policy where you work, knowing that this will lead to certain consequences. Other outcomes may be that you are considering a career move, or want to engage in further educational activity, and you need to work out the feasibility of the options available.

Summary

- 'What' questions help us to select an experience to write about reflectively by setting the parameters.
- They help us to identify the experience, frame the purpose and consider the consequences of writing about a particular event.

Activity

This activity is going to run through all six of the 5WH cues to help you to select an experience that will form the basis of some reflective writing in the next chapter. These are the basis, however, for any reflective activity that you do. It is worth doing this on paper, in note form, to act as a guide for your writing about the event.

First, identify an experience at work that has happened in the past five days. Then work through the 'what' questions above.

'Why' questions

'Why' questions help us to establish the importance of spending time reflecting on a particular incident, and the significance of it for us.

- Why am I reflecting on this? This asks us to frame the experience within our practice and to justify it as worthy of reflection over and above other experiences. This maybe because it fits criteria for student assessment or key targets for service delivery. It may, though, have a whole range of reasons such as:
  — contributing to a portfolio of evidence
  — exploring alternatives to courses of actions
  — enabling a solution to a problem
  — facilitating learning
  — contributing to appraisal

- Why is this experience important? Try to establish the significance of the experience for you.

Activity

Using the experience you have identified, ask yourself the 'why' questions.

'When' questions

'When' questions help us to plan the timing of our reflective activity by asking us about the urgency of reflection. They link closely with the 'how' and 'who' questions because they are about the environment and strategy for reflection, rather than the processes.

- When can you explore it more thoroughly? Some experiences are amenable to reflection immediately after they have happened. Others may benefit from waiting, for instance when they have resulted in an emotional reaction, or when the consequences of the event mean that immediate action needs to occur, such as in patient emergencies. You may also need to consider the context in which you will be reflecting, such as whether this is done within clinical supervision, appraisal, assessment, tutorials, etc.
- When do I need to resolve it? Again, some events have immediate requirements, but others can wait for reflective activity to occur. Not all things need to be dealt with on the spot, and for many, a 24-hour cooling off period, when events may look different, may bring less subjective reflection and a better resolution.
- When do I need to take action? This question follows on from the previous ones, and can help you to make a decision about when the reflective activity needs to happen.

Activity

Now answer the three 'when' questions.

'Where' questions

If reflection on action is to be effective it needs to be given time and space and commitment. Clearly, finding both the emotional and physical space where you will be uninterrupted is not easy in a busy working shift, and you may need to commit to doing this in your own time and away from the workplace. If you are choosing to reflect with others, you clearly need to take them into consideration and fit the 'where' into their needs as well. It may be that reflection takes place in another person's office, in the staff room, or in another quiet room; it can just as easily take place in a coffee bar as in a more formal place.

If you are going to write reflectively, you may need to be near a computer or to have a desk to write at. Other people are happy writing in informal locations – on the way home on public transport, at a café or even in bed.

Activity

Now answer the 'where' questions.

'Who' questions

'Who' questions ask you to decide whether you want to reflect alone or with others, and to consider the benefits and disadvantages of both.

These questions also raise the issues of whether you will need to ask the consent of others, such as patients, to record reflective activity, and of confidentiality.

Similarly, your reflective outcomes may have consequences for other people.

Activity

Who do you want to reflect with? Why?
Who do you need to gain consent from?
Who might be affected by the outcomes, or future action you may take?

'How' questions

Finally, we reach the 'how' questions, which relate to the strategies you will adopt when reflecting.

- How can I reflect most effectively? Consider whether to reflect alone or with others; verbally, in my head or in writing; using a framework or creating my own cue questions; recording the reflection in some way or not.
- How can I learn from this incident? This question asks for a commitment to the activity and its outcomes. If you are not prepared to follow the reflective processes through into action, you may need to reconsider whether this is the right experience to be reflecting on at this time.

Activity

Now complete the 5WH cues using the 'how' questions.

Summary

- These cues help us to explore the reasons behind the choice of experience to reflect on.
- They enable us to establish the context of both the reflective activity and the circumstances under which we will reflect.

These cues cover a range of activities, from enabling you to reflect on the spot to framing questions about developing the event further and identifying strategies for later reflection. The Institute for Reflective Practice (irp_uk@btopenworld.com) together with medical educators at Northampton General Hospital has devised an innovative way of facilitating reflection with junior doctors using credit-card sized record cards that are filled in throughout the working day, recording an incident and an immediate reaction to it. These are then developed more fully, resulting in an A4 written action plan arising from the incident. This strategy enables the doctor to reflect using whatever processes they find most suitable and appropriate for them, but ensures that there is evidence of their development and action taken within the professional portfolio of their development. This strategy safeguards the writer from concerns about the content of the documents in terms of litigation and the Data Protection Act 1998 (see Chapter 8 for further information on this). It also means that the internal and personal reflective processes of the practitioner are not available for public scrutiny, thus creating an element of personal safety.

Borton's framework

However, a simpler one, and one that is therefore easier to remember, is Borton's (1970) framework. This latter framework has the advantage that it doesn't draw the practitioner down particular lines of questioning and therefore frees them to focus their activity where they want to use it. Borton identified three question stems:

- what?
- so what?
- now what?

The job of the reflector is to complete the question according to what they want to achieve from the reflective activity. So, for instance, 'what' questions may be:

- What happened here?
- What did I do?
- What was I feeling?
- What did others do?
- What were the consequences of these actions?

This provides a descriptive stage (stages one and two of the reflective processes), but in a shorthand version that enables the practitioner to focus on the key issues of the incident. These are the ones that spring to mind when thinking about an event, and are therefore uppermost in the mind – helpful in thoughtful reflection. This summary then becomes the focus for reflection on action by moving to Borton's next set of questions – those initiated by 'so what', such as:

- So what was I trying to achieve?
- So what were my decision processes at the time?
- So what knowledge or evidence was I using to inform my decisions?
- So what don't I know and need to find out?
- So what could I have done differently?

These take the practitioner through reflective stages three, four and five, enabling them to consider their knowledge, skill and experience base, as well as exploring their decisions and actions and weighing them against possible alternatives. Borton then moves onto the 'now what' questions, such as:

- Now what more do I need to know?
- Now what needs to change?
- Now what action do I need to take?

It is difficult to carry a framework in your head, but the relative simplicity of Borton's work does provide a starting point and is easy to remember once you have the hang of it. It does have its disadvantages, however, in that you could be tempted into superficial reflection and in only focusing on issues you want to address, as opposed to those that might be a bit more challenging or uncomfortable to explore. By being dependent upon the practitioner in completing the questions it is easy to remain in the same thought processes that we always use, to avoid difficult areas for you and not be challenged out of these. Working with another person, such as a colleague or clinical supervisor, helps to avoid this problem.

Whilst the idea of carrying a framework around in your head is an attractive one, in reality we are less likely to structure the reflective activity that goes on in our heads. Individual reflection of this sort is more likely to be reflection in action that is unconscious and draws on the knowledge base we already have in order to inform our current practice. This will not lead to change and development unless it moves into our consciousness and facilitates reflection-on-action. This is likely to be more effective if it moves beyond staying in our heads and is given voice in some other way.

Summary

- Reflecting by yourself has two main forms – thoughtful reflection that goes on in your head, and written reflection.

- Frameworks and models can be used to guide your individual reflective activity.
- Choosing a simple, easy to remember framework will be most effective.
- Thoughtful reflection tends to be unstructured and therefore less likely to result in new perspectives.

Developing critical thinking

Key to developing skills as a reflective practitioner is the development of critical thinking as you develop throughout your professional career. Critical thinking is one of the ways in which practitioners make decisions about their practice. It has been defined as 'the process of purposeful, self-regulatory judgement and interactive reflective reasoning process' (Facione *et al.* 1994 p. 345). Critical thinkers are:

- habitually inquisitive
- trustful of reason
- flexible
- honest in facing personal biases
- willing to reconsider
- orderly in complex matters
- well informed
- open-minded
- fair minded in evaluations
- prudent in making judgements
- clear about issues
- diligent in seeking relevant information
- reasonable in the selection of criteria focused in enquiry
- persistent in seeking results that are as precise as the subject and circumstances of enquiry permit. (American Philosophical Association 1990)

Activity

Assess yourself against the APA's characteristics of critical thinkers.

Where are your strengths?
Where do you think you need to develop further?

Reflective practice requires practitioners to develop high levels of critical thinking, particularly as they move towards independence in their practice and are required to be able to justify their decision-making and be accountable for their practice in law. This means having an explicit awareness of the ways in which you arrive at your decisions and being prepared to debate and defend them with others.

Reflecting by yourself, and thinking reflectively is undoubtedly contributory to the development of critical thinking and reflective practice, but it is limited in terms of the depth of reflection that happens and the extent to which it can help you take a different perspective. There are two ways in which you can choose to develop your reflective skills so that they are more effective: by writing reflectively, or by reflecting with other people.

Summary

- Critical thinking is central to successful reflective practice.
- The attributes of critical thinkers have been identified and can be worked towards by practitioners developing reflective skills.

Using others to help your reflective activity

There are many benefits to enlisting others in your reflective work:

- They bring a fresh pair of eyes to a situation.
- They can take an objective stance.
- They can ask the questions we won't ask ourselves and stimulate deeper reflection.
- They may offer different perspectives on events.
- They can act as a sounding board for our ideas.
- They may validate our thoughts.
- They may put events in a different context and put events in different political and social frames.
- They contribute to our understanding from a different knowledge and skills base.
- They may suggest alternative courses of action. (Adapted from Jasper 2003 pp. 174–179.)

Working with others is undoubtedly risky; you are choosing to share your thoughts and open yourself up to someone else's gaze. Therefore it is important to be very clear about the parameters of a reflective relationship with another person. The context of the relationship may differ. Here are a few that I have encountered:

- clinical supervision (see Chapter 7 for more on this)
- appraisal, personal development or independent performance review in the workplace
- working with an assessor, mentor or academic tutor for the purpose of learning
- peer review or buddying in the workplace
- one to one with another person
- team development
- group or peer work in a classroom setting

- working with a 'critical friend' outside your immediate workplace
- peer/colleague support in a study group
- a friend or relative outside the working context.

For reflective activity with others to be effective it is important to establish the ground rules of the relationship or encounter before starting. Fundamental to this is the emotional safety of the people concerned and of the reflector in particular. It is worth talking these issues through, before you get together if possible, to ensure that you are both coming to the meeting with the same expectations, clarity about each other's role and the purpose of the meeting.

It is also worth thinking about the following guidance for those doing the listening and supporting in the relationship:

- Be positive and supportive.
- Think about the language you use when responding to and facilitating other's reflection; try not to criticise or use negative language.
- Comment on the content or the reflection, not the person. This is especially so when written accounts form the focus of the work.
- Agree on confidentiality, or otherwise, in order to provide safety for participants to say what they feel and think.
- Establish boundaries of trust.
- The reflective practitioner can make clear the focus or parameters of the issues before they start.
- Make clear at the start the criteria for assessment if this is part of the process.

These need to be considered within the context of the relationship between the reflector and the listener; where there is a managerial relationship, or the reflective work is part of assessment processes or supervising, the stance of the listener may be different. However, to get the most out of reflecting with others, it is important for the reflector to feel safe in exposing their own actions and feelings, and therefore the purpose of the reflective activity (as a learning tool) needs to be paramount in the listener's mind. Their role is one of active support in facilitating the reflective processes for the reflector; it is not, on the whole, appropriate for the listener to be critical or judgemental. A skilful facilitator will enable the reflector to come to their own conclusions and judgements.

Activity

What might be the risks of reflecting with other people?

The risks you identified here are all likely to contribute to the creation of barriers within the reflective relationship, resulting in the activity being less than effective. These might relate to:

- feeling judged
- the language that others use
- negative body language
- you not liking the 'reflected' self
- feeling talked about outside the group/relationship
- feeling criticised, and your professional practice being questioned.

When these happen, true reflection is unlikely to occur.

Central to Gillie Bolton's (2005) approach to professional development through reflective writing is group critical discussions of narrative writing of various forms – stories, poems, etc. This has the benefit of enabling critique from the differing multi-professional viewpoints of others, as well as facilitating the critical thinking of the person concerned.

Summary

- Reflecting with others expands the reflector's horizons by widening the reflective gaze beyond the individual.
- The reflective relationship needs to be negotiated and clear parameters and ground rules established prior to the reflective activity.
- Reflection with others can take place between pairs or in larger groups.

Chapter summary

In this chapter I have introduced both the underpinnings of reflective practice and some ways in which this may be achieved. As nursing practice increases in complexity, as nurses progress to truly independent practice as specialists and consultants, and as nurses build their contribution as equal members within the inter-professional health care team, it becomes increasingly important that nurses develop as reflective practitioners able to account for and justify the decisions they make in practice. Becoming a reflective practitioner involves learning and practising reflective skills, just as learning clinical competence takes years of formal and experiential learning. Building strategies for reflective practice is a journey, which involves starting with an awareness of the basic skills and techniques, and an understanding of the process and purpose of these, and developing into the underpinning ways of working that ensure safe and competent practice, which develops and changes in response to new understandings and knowledge.

References

American Philosophical Association (1990) *Critical Thinking: a Statement of Expert Consensus for Purposes of Educational Assessment and Instruction: The Delphi Report: Research Findings and Recommendations Prepared for the Committee on Pre-college Philosophy.* American Philosophical Society, Millbrae, CA.

Atkins, S. and Murphy, K. (1994) Reflective Practice. *Nursing Standard,* **8** (39), 49–56.

Benner, P. (1984) *From Novice to Expert.* Addison-Wesley, CA.

Bolton, G. (2005) *Reflective Practice – Writing and Professional Development* (2nd edn). Sage, London.

Borton, T. (1970) *Reach, Touch and Teach.* Hutchinson, London.

Boud, D., Keogh, R. and Walker, D. (1985) *Reflection: Turning Learning into Experience.* Paul Chapman Publishing, London.

Boyd, E.M. and Fales, A.W. (1983) Reflective learning: key to learning from experience. *Journal of Humanistic Psychology,* **23** (2), 99–117.

Bulman, C. (2004) An introduction to reflection. In: Chapter one in Bulman, C. and Schutz. S. (eds) *Reflective Practice in Nursing* (3rd edn). Blackwell Publishing, Oxford.

Department of Health (2001) National Service Framework for Diabetes: Standards. HMSO, London.

Dewey, J. (1938) *Experience and Education.* Macmillan, New York.

Facione, P.A., Facione, N.C. and Sanchez, C.A. (1994) Critical thinking disposition as a measure of competent clinical judgement: the development of the California Critical Thinking Dispositional Inventory. *Journal of Nursing Education,* **33**, 345–350.

Gibbs, G. (1988) *Learning by Doing. A Guide to Teaching and Learning Methods.* Further Education Unit, Oxford Polytechnic, Oxford.

Goodman, J. (1984) Reflection and teacher education: a case study and theoretical analysis. *Interchanges,* **15**, 9–26.

Holm, D. and Stephenson, S. (1994) Reflection – a student's perspective. In: Palmer, A., Burns, S. and Bulman, C. (eds) *Reflective Practice in Nursing.* Blackwell Publishing, Oxford.

Institute for Reflective Practice irp_uk@btopenworld.com

Jasper, M. (2003) *Beginning Reflective Practice.* Nelson Thornes, Cheltenham.

Johns, C. (1998) Opening the doors of perception. In: Johns, C. and Freshwater, D. (eds) *Transforming Nursing Through Reflective Practice,* pp. 1–20. Blackwell Publishing, Oxford.

Johns, C. (2004) *Becoming a Reflective Practitioner* (2nd edn). Blackwell Publishing, Oxford.

Kim, S.H. (1999) Critical reflective inquiry for knowledge development in nursing practice. *Journal of Advanced Nursing,* **29**, (5), 1205–1212.

Kolb, D. (1984) *Experiential Learning as the Science of Learning and Development.* Prentice Hall, Englewood Cliffs, NJ.

Mezirow, J. (1981) A critical theory of adult learning and education. *Adult Education*, **32** (1), 3–24.

Nursing and Midwifery Council (2004) *Code of Professional Conduct: Standards for Conduct, Performance and Ethics*. NMC, London.

Rolfe, G., Freshwater, D. and Jasper, M. (2001) *Critical Reflection for Nursing and the Helping Professions: a User's Guide*. Palgrave, Basingstoke.

Schön, D. (1983) *The Reflective Practitioner*. Temple Smith, London.

Reflective writing for professional development

Reflective writing in professional development

Writing brings with it the feature of permanency; it exists until someone decides to throw it away or delete it from a computer. Writing is therefore an essential adjunct for documenting our professional development and to provide evidence to demonstrate our continuing and developing competence as practitioners.

In practice professions, however, writing is not noted as being a strong feature of professional practice. Whilst there is research writing, writing clinical records and writing reports, practitioners tend not to have a culture of writing about their practice or, indeed, about themselves. However, the PREP (NMC 2004a) requirements for triennial registration for nurses brought with them the need for nurses to have a documented record of their professional development over a three-year period, available for audit purposes if requested. This puts a responsibility on the nurse for, at the minimum, keeping a paper record, together with evidence, that supports their claim to have met the continuing professional development requirements. The use of portfolios and evidence is developed further in Chapter 6. What I want to explore in this chapter, however, is how reflective writing can be used as part of a practitioner's practice in contributing to their decision-making and their professional development. In addition, reflective writing helps us to understand ourselves, and our experiences better, and will often enable us to resolve issues as a result.

To do this, I will first look at the nature of writing, and reflective writing, as tools for development in their own right, rather than as tools for simply recording and documenting. I will then continue to build on the previous chapter in exploring micro-methods for written reflection. Finally, I will present a model of how experienced nurses use reflective writing within portfolios to demonstrate their accountability for their practice, and show how this links to professional development.

Activity

Take a few minutes to think about the features of writing.

What makes it what it is?
How is it different from speaking and just thinking?
How do you know how to do it?
Do you need any special skills to do it?
What do you use writing for?
Are there times when you would choose to write something, as opposed to just thinking or saying it?
How do you feel about writing yourself, especially in relation to using it by yourself as part of your professional development?

The nature of writing

We all write (we have to) as a primary means of communication within our society. As a professional practitioner we write mainly to record our or others' actions and to pass on information to our colleagues. We create permanent records about our patients that are depended upon by others as a basis for future action and treatment. Records may also by used in a court of law as evidence, and are therefore subjected to certain rules and strategies to ensure that they are sound and effective (NMC 2005) (record-keeping as a feature of professional practice will be covered in more detail in Chapter 8). To function in practice, therefore, we need to have sophisticated writing skills to ensure that our communication is effective, intelligible and accurate. We need to learn to use the rules and features of writing to enable us to function effectively as practitioners.

Writing has its own features:

- It is a purposeful activity; you don't write by mistake.
- It is a private activity, until and unless you make the results public.
- Writing has its own sets of rules: language, words, spelling, grammar, syntax, punctuation, which help the writer to make sense of their thoughts.
- Private writing may decide to ignore these rules; the writing only needs to make sense and have meaning to the writer.
- It is a way of ordering your thoughts.
- It creates a permanent record; it is there until you decide to destroy it.
- It helps to make contact with unexamined thoughts and create unique connections between them and new ideas.
- It draws on previously forgotten memories and knowledge.
- It provides focus to your mental activity, helping to structure your thoughts.
- It facilitates creativity, allowing us to develop ideas in increasing complexity.

We use all of these features every working day to ensure that our professional practice is documented and that patients receive continuity in care that is safe. Within professional development though, they are useful as both a process and an end result in helping us to get to where we want to be, and record the effects.

Reflective writing is a particular form of writing:

- It is done for the purposes of learning.
- It enables a deeper and more complete understanding of a subject, event or experience.
- It may result in practice and professional development and contribute to decision-making.
- It is experiential; it arises from the past, from your knowledge and skills base, your professional experiences and from your life as a human being in the world.
- It can adopt a range of strategies, from lacking structure in creative techniques, to a tight structure in analytical techniques.

- It may be organised through the stages of the reflective processes.
- It provides a way of exploring a range of issues from different perspectives.
- It enables the connection of disparate sets of information and data, which result in the creation of practice-based knowledge unique to the individual.
- It provides a way of exploring issues of which you are aware but may not want to acknowledge or deal with.

Reflective writing also provides a tangible artefact that you may use to:

- store in a portfolio as evidence of professional development
- result in an action plan
- discuss with someone else
- use in clinical supervision
- contribute to your personal development plan
- discuss at your appraisal
- submit for assessment purposes.

Summary

- Writing has a set of defining features which can be used in professional development and reflection as both a process and an end result.
- Reflective writing is a specific form of writing aimed at helping us to learn from our experiences.
- Reflective writing helps us to understand what has happened to us in the past and to take a new perspective on it.
- Reflective writing provides a permanent record of our development that can be used as an artefact for several purposes.

Activity

How does reflective writing differ from the writing that you have done previously?

Can you identify any experiences from your past that would benefit writing about in this way?

When to write

There are two main sub-questions within this question. First is the question of when you choose to write about an event reflectively as opposed to exploring it in a different way, such as with a colleague, within clinical supervision, or by musing on it by yourself at a quiet time. Taking the decision to use an experience as the basis of reflective writing means that it is stuck in your head for some reason; often this is because it is unresolved and is making you feel uncomfortable in some way. However, experiences stand out in our minds for a reason, and warrant writing about if they:

- won't go away
- are preventing you from moving on in a relationship with another person
- arise from a knowledge or skill deficit
- arise from witnessing poor professional practice or issues regarding safe practice
- may be difficult if shared with others before being resolved in your own mind
- contravene your own ethical or moral values base
- went exceptionally well and made you feel happy about yourself
- involved new or different experiences that may lead to new learning and understanding.

Reflective writing involves exploring an issue in depth. It takes a commitment of time and energy and therefore the writer needs to know that the results will be worthwhile and it is good use of their time before starting on it. Using reflective writing selectively, to explore issues that are deep-rooted and less amenable to other forms of reflection, ensures that this becomes part of your reflective strategies, and is used purposefully, rather than as a paper exercise only.

Second is the question of creating the physical and emotional space to write; this is often the greatest barrier to writing, whether real or used as an excuse for not writing. For some people, the only way of starting to resolve issues is to write about them in the first instance. These may be issues that you are aware of, but often, as Gillie Bolton (2005) suggests, they surface as a result of sitting down and beginning to write. She provides several examples of the spontaneous generation of issues for practitioners that then became the focus for reflective exploration. Her techniques, which she calls 'through the looking glass', are worth reading if you want to know more about generating material that can be used as the basis of both reflecting with others and for more personal and individual work. Other ways of generating reflective events are to:

- jot key events in a day down as the day progresses
- make a point of reviewing the day, in a couple of minutes before you go off duty
- summarise, with another person how your morning/day/week has gone

- write down new experiences
- review a particular event
- identify a situation that you handled well/badly
- explore a situation where you felt you needed more knowledge
- explore a situation which could have had several different solutions.

However, we can all find ways of avoiding writing, especially if it was not a part of your professional education when you were a student. Writing in many forms is done on a daily basis by all professionals; reflective writing doesn't tend to be one of these. Reflective writing means taking a conscious decision to spend some private time away from others, doing this in preference to other things that you could be doing, and to commit this time to your professional development. Many practitioners have, in the past, seen practice as what they do as part of their paid work time, as opposed to something they commit their own time to. However, the parameters of professional practice are clear, as are the requirements of the NMC, in that professional practitioners are expected to engage in lifelong learning which might necessitate using their own time.

Another issue is the physical requirement for writing. For many people, this means using a computer or other technical device, such as a palm-held unit or even a mobile phone. These might need you to be in a certain fixed place in order to write, or to have access to electricity or a phone line. Other people prefer to write onto paper, which may be more flexible in terms of the physical space needed and the time which can be committed to it. For instance, using public transport affords time that can be used for writing. Using travelling time in this way also brings the bonus of time-limiting your writing. If, for instance, you know that your journey will take ten minutes, you can set yourself an eight-minute limit for writing a description of an event. This enables you to focus on the main features of the event because you know you have to get to the end before your train pulls in. This will then provide you with a description of key points that you can then work on later. Another way to use short periods of time is by using the 'three a day' technique explained below. Finally, concentration is needed to write reflectively, as your thoughts need to be given free rein to drift in ways that they could not do if your thoughts are divided or there are competing demands on your time.

Summary

- Within reflective activity, decisions need to be made about what experiences are worthy of writing about reflectively.
- Reflective writing necessitates a commitment to finding both physical space and the time to reflect effectively.

Activity

Finding time to write within a busy life is not easy. Most people would say, when asked, that they are always busy and don't have any free time to fit anything else in.

Perhaps then, the trick is to review what you do, and the ways in which you spend your time, and see whether you can reorganise your time to fit other things in. Again, this activity will take time if you feel you need the space to do it in one go. But, another way of doing it is to question, throughout the next week, why you are doing the things you are doing as you are doing them.

For instance, do you really have to do the dusting/cleaning/ironing, etc.? What will happen if you don't do these things? Does it really matter if that happens? Is there anyone else who can share in these tasks? Can the children get their own packed lunch, tidy their rooms, put their clothes away or do their own washing and ironing? One hour per week is not a lot to find. For women especially, our time is often committed to doing things for others, often as routine, or because others like it that way. Finding time for yourself, if it means enabling others to take more responsibility for their own welfare, can actually also be seen as a selfless act and bring you benefits at the same time.

Structuring reflective writing

Any of the frameworks introduced in Chapter 2 can be used to write reflectively. These provide a useful way of working through an issue without the reflector having to create the strategy they are going to use. The frameworks may enable questions to be asked that you may not, or do not, want to think about. Selecting different frameworks to work through issues, which arise from alternative values and beliefs, will stimulate you to take another perspective to experiences you have had. However, it is not essential to use a formal structure for your writing, and it may be that you prefer to write, sometimes, using free-flowing text.

Using the 5WH cues

The flexibility of the 5WH cues enables us to focus our reflective activity to our particular needs at the time. Initially, these are about the selection of the event itself and working out the purpose and possible outcomes we want to achieve as a result. If you have worked through the activity on selecting an experience to reflect on in Chapter 2 you will already have arrived at something to reflect about. If not, have a look at these again to ensure you know, but focus this on written reflection, rather than another type:

- what you want to write about
- why you want to write about it
- when you will do the writing
- where you will do the writing
- who else is likely to be involved
- how you might want to write.

Using the 5WH cues at this stage can therefore be focused on the reflective processes themselves. Table 3.1 provides examples of questions that might be asked to guide reflective writing as well as any other sort of reflective activity that might happen.

Table 3.1   Using the 5WH cues to guide reflection.

What	Why
happened? did I do? did others do? was I feeling? was the result? went well? went unexpectedly? went badly? am I worried about? is my responsibility? is my part in the experience? might be the consequences? was the knowledge I was using? did I learn? do I need to know? skills do I need to develop?	did it happen? did I act/think/feel this way? is it significant/important?
When	**Where**
did it happen? am I going to take action? will I revisit my reflections?	did it happen?
Who	**How**
was involved? might be affected? needs to know? needs to take action?	did it happen? can I learn from it? can I take a different perspective? can I resolve the situation? can I prevent it happening again?

Summary

- There are no rules for structuring your reflective writing.
- Published frameworks and models may be used to guide your reflective writing.
- You may prefer to use a strategy that is less rigid and adaptable to your own learning and professional development activities.

Activity

Do you usually use a structure for your reflective writing?
If so, why?
What would happen if you used a less/more structured approach?
Are you willing to try?

Strategies for reflective writing

Strategies for reflective writing fall into two main groups – analytical strategies and creative strategies (Rolfe *et al.* 2001; Jasper 2003). However, in many ways these can be seen as two ends of a continuum, with the different types of strategy spread along the continuum. This is shown in Figure 3.1.

Analytical strategies tend to be used when someone else is likely to see your writing, such as when you are using it within an assignment or when it will go into a portfolio. Analytical strategies use the full range of the reflective processes to complete the ERA cycle to ensure that conclusions are reached and action is framed. They often follow

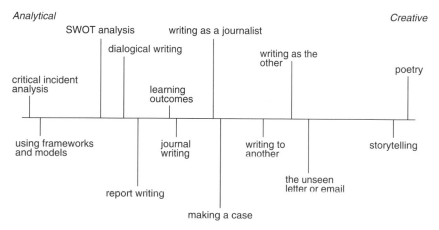

Figure 3.1 Strategies for reflective writing.

frameworks or models, but, as they move across the continuum, they may become more free-flowing in their style. Fuller descriptions of techniques at this end of the continuum are summarised in Table 3.2.

In contrast, creative strategies may stop at the descriptive phase and not progress through any of the analytical stages of the reflective processes. They may also be used to provide a trigger for discussion with others, such as in clinical supervision, discussions with a mentor, or in group reflective sessions. You may also use them in order to capture one version of an event, in a colourful or descriptive way that would not happen if you were using an analytical strategy. These strategies are often used to get past the initial emotional response to something that has happened to us, such as anger, hurt, embarrassment, insult, outrage, inadequacy, sadness, disbelief and grief.

The selection of either of these strategies for reflecting on a particular incident will depend on a number of things, including the emotional reaction you had to the incident itself and the feelings you are left with at this moment in time. Some of the criteria you might want to consider when selecting a strategy for reflective writing are:

- The stimulus for writing: are you choosing to write spontaneously, or are you doing it for a course requirement, in preparation for group work or clinical supervision, for instance?
- Who is likely to see it? Will this be purely private writing, or will it be seen by others?
- The nature of the incident: was it something that has personal implications for you, or is it a more remote experience (this may stimulate you to think about whether it is personal or professional development that you are engaging in).
- What do you want the outcome to be?
- Who else may be involved?
- Are there any professional or ethical issues that may arise?

Ultimately, although you will be writing in order to learn from your experiences, you need to bear in mind that different outcomes will result from different strategies selected, or from different models or frameworks used. Therefore, it is worth spending some time considering the selection of the strategies you will use, as you are going to devote considerable time to writing reflectively and you want it to produce tangible results at the end. Often, our inability to move on from an event results from the way we look at it. Just with any other way of working, we develop habits and routines that keep us within our 'comfort zone'. Although routines are useful in maintaining our well-being, they can also prevent us from seeing things in a different way, or taking a different perspective on an event. In short, routines help us to see the world from a position of stability and safety. However, sometimes we need to challenge ourselves to move beyond the routines and this comfort zone, so that we can develop. Choosing

Table 3.2 Features of reflective writing strategies.

Strategy	Features
Analytical strategies	
Critical incident analysis	An event is 'critical' if it stands out in some way and can be described in its entirety
	Establishes the important features of an event
	Aimed at identifying successful and unsuccessful behaviours or features
Frameworks and models	Uses a predetermined framework
	Underpinned by a set of beliefs and values
	Takes a staged approach
	Works methodically through the stages
	Works towards desired outcomes
Dialogical writing	The writer engages in a dialogue with themselves
	The next question arises from the answer to the previous one
	Issues arise during and as a result of the analysis
Report writing	Key and objective features only are reported
	Tends not to include analysis of emotions
	Lacks subjectivity
Writing as a journalist	Takes an outsider's approach to an event
	Aims at objectivity and giving weighting to different elements
Making a case	Argues from a particular viewpoint
	May present two sides to a case
	May incorporate underpinning knowledge and evidence
	Similar to an academic writing style
Journal keeping	Compiled on an incremental basis
	Provides a record of events and experiences
	Focuses on identifying learning or experience
	Can contain a range of elements, including reflective reviews
SWOT analysis	Uses headings: strengths, weaknesses, opportunities and threats (or barriers)
	Focuses reflection through evaluating real and potential elements
Creative strategies	
Writing to another	Focuses on retelling the main features or elements of an experience
	Can take differing perspectives depending on who the imaginary recipient is
	Acts as a way of freeing the mind from the emotional content so the essential features of the experience can be further worked on
Writing as the other	Enables the writer to see things from the other person's viewpoint
	Forces the writer to distance themselves from their own viewpoint
The unseen letter or email	This is a tension-relieving strategy, allowing the writer to pour everything onto paper and rid themselves of emotional baggage
	It focuses on the subjective experience of the writer and their feelings
	Under no circumstances should this be sent

Continued

Table 3.2 *Continued*

Strategy	Features
Storytelling/fantasy	To some extent, all descriptive records are 'stories' Framing the experience as a story enables the writer to view it as one version of something; there may be several other, equally valid versions Using different names for people helps to use the experience as a story
Poetry	This strategy reduces the experience to its essential, and most important elements, for the writer The imposition of cadence, order and structure used in creating poetry, redefines the elements

to use a reflective strategy that you wouldn't normally be comfortable with may be the first step to enlightenment.

Summary

- Two main strategies for reflective writing have been identified – analytical strategies and creative strategies.
- Analytical strategies tend to be more structured and are used when others are involved in the reflective process.
- Creative strategies tend to be used for helping people to get through incidents where strong emotions have occurred.
- There are a wide range of strategies available across this continuum, all of which are valuable in the nurse's 'kitbag' for reflection.
- These strategies enable nurses to find different ways of perceiving events and help them to move beyond familiar ways of thinking.

Activity

Consider the variety of strategies presented in this section. Give each of them a score, 1–10, of how attractive they are to you and whether you would be likely to use them yourself. One would be 'not at all likely'; ten would be 'very likely'.
Now ask yourself why it is you scored them in this way.

Techniques for reflective writing

There are many, many techniques that can be used for reflection – too many to try to cover in this chapter. Any of the books in the reference list (for this chapter and Chapter 2) will provide more help with specific techniques, such as the use of the frameworks and models. In this section, therefore, I just want to cover some ideas for getting started in reflective writing, for generating material to be used as the basis of reflection, and for developing that further within the notion of personal and professional development.

First of all, choosing a strategy for reflection may be the only stimulus that is needed, as many of these will take you down a particular route. For instance, writing a reflective log or keeping a journal may help you to develop a writing habit from relatively small beginnings. Making a case for a change in practice may lead onto further practice developments that you had not previously envisaged, which in turn may lead to a role or job change.

Short-period techniques/stimulatory/getting started techniques

These techniques are about making the most of opportunities for reflective writing in the short and immediate term. One of the barriers to reflective writing is seen to be the apparent time commitment needed for it. These techniques are all ones that can be used on a day-to-day basis and are not really additional to your work. They enable you to make a note of experiences as they occur, or very soon after, so that you can then go on to use them in a more reflective exploratory way at a later date if you want to.

The three-a-day technique

This asks you to list the three most important things that have happened to you during your shift. The alternatives to this technique are legion; for instance, you could vary the focus of the technique by altering the subject such as the three things:

- you enjoyed most
- you enjoyed least
- you learnt during the day
- that challenged you the most
- you didn't know
- you felt confident about
- you felt inadequate doing
- that went well
- that didn't go as planned.

The list is as long as your imagination, but what you find will happen is that the things that come into your mind are the things that are most important. You may then choose to explore these in greater depth at a later time. It is worth carrying a small notebook to use for this sort of work, as it will provide you with a reminder and a record of the issues that came to mind.

The credit card technique

This is so-called for two reasons: first, because using cards the shape of credit cards is a convenient way of carrying notes of our experiences, which can be built upon at a later date. Second, you will be storing up 'credit' in the form of key things that happen to you during a day that act as an aide-memoire for when you have space to reflect by yourself, or with other people. I first came across this idea at a conference run by the Institute of Reflective Practice (www.reflectivepractices.co.uk), where it was introduced as a way of enabling junior doctors to store up experiences as a focus for reflective activity (Jeffrey 2006). The cards developed for these doctors tap into reflection in action (Schön 1983), asking for on-the-spot recording of an immediate experience, almost as it happens. There are boxes to record the focus for reflection (using cues), links with the General Medical Council's principles and the immediate responses of the doctor (again, using cues). The doctors are then encouraged to reflect after the event, in private, on a single sheet of paper, confining their writing to learning about themselves, action to be taken, suggested discussion topics and alterations to their personal development plan. If the doctor wishes to write more, in terms of their reflective strategy, they do so in the certain knowledge that it will be private, and not required to be made public. This technique is subject to copyright at present, and can therefore only be presented in these broad terms. However, the basic, simple principles can be developed and adapted for any practitioner in creating their own record cards and focusing the cue questions on the particular aspects of exploring their experiences that will result in their own learning and professional development.

Time-limited stimuli

Gillie Bolton (2005) uses this technique to generate material for group reflective activity, followed by individual reflective writing away from the group. The idea is to set a short period of time, such as six minutes, within which you write about whatever comes into your head. This is a difficult task initially, and certainly promotes scepticism when first suggested to people. However, the discipline of having to put something on paper in that time seems to stimulate the mind to drag key experiences from its depths to form the basis for reflection.

My day

Another technique is to provide a brief summary of your day, highlighting the key elements using cues devised by yourself. Although similar to the three-a-day technique, this provides an overview of the day and can be as long, or short, as you want to make it. For some, this will mean compiling a log of the whole day; others may focus on just one event. Other strategies are to focus on listing the skills you have used, or the patients you have seen; the other members of the multidisciplinary team you have worked with, or perhaps the sources of knowledge or evidence you have used to inform your practice. Once identified, these again can be used within the reflective processes as a stimulus for your later reflective activity.

The NMC *Code of Professional Conduct*
As the foundations for professional practice, the clauses in the *Code of Professional Conduct* (NMC 2004b) can be used to focus reflective writing. Each one of the clauses draws attention to different aspects of practice. By reviewing your recent experiences and exploring them against one of the clauses you will generate evidence of your continuing professional development as well as your accountability for your practice within the code.

Activity

Select two of these techniques, and spend a short period of time (such as five minutes) using each one to generate some topics for reflection. Write them down, and store them away for later use.

Summary

- Various techniques can be used to start or stimulate your written reflective activity.
- These range from keeping on-the-spot notes, to reviewing your day, to using external stimuli and structure such as the NMC *Code of Professional Conduct*.
- They all provide a way of capturing your everyday experiences as they happen.

Medium-term and developmental techniques

These really relate to making the most of the experiences you have in a planned and productive way. Look at the strategies in Table 3.2 again and decide which of these could be used within your own reflective writing. For instance, you may decide to keep a reflective log or journal that you contract with yourself to write in once a week (or more, or less). Similarly, you may decide that you will set aside a period of time each week to review what has happened and record your feelings and reflections. Another way to do this is to identify one event that stands out in your mind to explore in depth each week.

Exploring in depth means engaging in the reflective processes of analysis, taking a different perspective, synthesis and planning action that move you on from having provided a description of the event (return to Chapter 2 for a review of these if you need to). Whilst remembering and describing an event will start you on the road to understanding more about it, and in doing so may help you to see something differently, the full benefit of reflective learning will not occur unless you are prepared to delve deeper into the experience and challenge yourself to see it from another perspective.

This need take no longer than an hour per week, yet the benefits that will accrue will be worth a lot more than can be summarised in those hours:

- You will have created an ongoing record of your development.
- You will have identified your learning needs.
- You will have created your professional portfolio in an incremental way.
- You will have evidence of achieving your CPD standard required for re-registration with the NMC.
- You will have learnt from your experiences.
- You will have developed action plans arising from your experiences.
- You will have material which you can build upon in terms of practice development.
- You may have solved problems in practice that have been around for some time.
- You will have a greater understanding of the way you work as a professional.

This is all for just one hour a week. Valuing the things you do well, and your successes, identifying your own development, and having an active and proactive role helps to boost your morale and motivate your future practice. Just as going to the gym brings about a feel-good factor because of endorphin release, so does the emotional equivalent of reflective writing in a positive way. You may even find that reflective writing becomes a habit; that it is as essential to you as any other part of your practice such as record-keeping, keeping your knowledge base up to date or working within a multidisciplinary team.

Long-term techniques

Once you have started on the medium-term strategies you may find that they become engrained as the way you practice. It is obviously impossible to know how many nurses write reflectively as most do it in private and keep the products of their writing to themselves. One simple way of continuing your reflective writing is to return to writing you have already done and re-view it in the light of the passage of time and more experience. Another strategy is to set yourself a 'revisiting' date for any entry in your portfolio/journal and keep a list of these (this, of course, is only for the more organised and structured person) to stimulate the activity. However, this is really only an extension of the way you would plan a care plan or package, with built-in review dates, so, if this is part of your existing clinical practice it is only a small step to incorporating it into your reflective writing.

However, we do have some examples of writers who share their writing together with the strategies they use and their own personal involvement in this. Chris Johns (2002), for example, demonstrates the use of his ever developing model of structured reflection by illustrating it with his own experiences. Other examples are found in the nursing literature, both in the professional and academic journals.

Central to long-term strategies is the commitment that a nurse makes to dedicating time to reflective writing. If this commitment is not there, the writing will not happen. Reflective writing is not compulsory for practice, but it does enable the nurse to understand more about themselves and their practice, in addition to providing stimuli for change in practice and practice development, whether this remains at a personal level, has wider implications within the working environment, or is at a professional level.

One strategy that is pertinent to all professional practitioners, however, is the need to keep a professional portfolio. Portfolios are explored in more detail in Chapter 6, where you will find strategies for constructing a portfolio and suggestions for how they can be used within your practice. Reflective writing, as part of professional development, is an essential component of a portfolio. Thus, the final section of this chapter explores how some experienced nurses use written reflection in their portfolios to demonstrate their accountability as practitioners.

Summary

- Medium and long-term strategies for written reflection need to become part of the way in which a nurse practises.
- Reflective writing, like any other long-term strategy, needs motivation and commitment.
- Reflective writing is not compulsory, but it does enable nurses to develop their own understanding of their practice and has resultant effects within the working environment.

Activity

Consider the ways in which you use reflection and reflective writing as part of your practice at present.

Do you feel you are making the most of opportunities that arise in practice for experiential learning through reflective writing?
What would you need to do to maximise these opportunities?
Could you devote an hour a week to reflective writing?
Do you feel you would benefit, and have the motivation to do this?
Will you do it?

Experienced nurses' use of reflective writing in professional portfolios

In this section I will explore how experienced nurses use reflective writing within their portfolios to demonstrate their accountability as registered practitioners. A total of 37 nurses told me about the ways they use reflective writing, spontaneously, to maintain a record of their work which would satisfy the NMC's requirements for triennial registration (Jasper 2006, submitted for publication).

Whilst demonstrating accountability was clearly the main factor in writing reflectively in their portfolios, the nurses identified four other key elements that resulted from reflective writing:

- their own professional development
- their personal development
- the development of their critical thinking abilities
- outcomes for (clinical) practice.

These will all be discussed in further detail in the sections below.

The main conclusions to be drawn from this study are that when reflective writing is embraced by practitioners as a chosen strategy and is used dynamically within their professional practice, it proves a useful and creative way of learning through experience. This results in the nurses having collected together a body of evidence, together with reflective reviews of their practice that demonstrates their professional accountability. Moreover the learning achieved is reflected back into practice development and improved care for patients, thus contributing to improved patient outcomes.

Summary

- Reflective writing used spontaneously and deliberately by nurses within their portfolios is aimed at developing a body of knowledge to demonstrate their professional accountability.
- This has four components: professional development, personal development, critical thinking and outcomes for (clinical) practice.

Demonstrating accountability through reflective writing

The way the four elements fit together to contribute to nurses being able to demonstrate their accountability is shown in Figure 3.2.

Whilst the core category (demonstrating accountability) presents the overall *raison d'être* for reflective writing within the portfolios, distinction is made between the outcomes of the reflective writing and the processes that are involved in it. Hence, personal and professional development, and outcomes for (clinical) practice are the results of

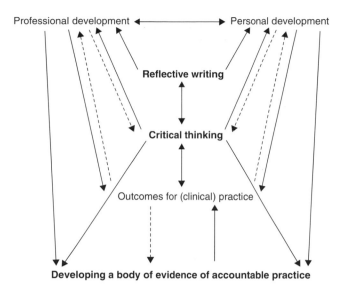

Figure 3.2 Jasper's (2004) model of experienced nurses' use of reflective writing in portfolios. Reproduced with permission from Bulman, C. and Schutz, S. (ed.) *Reflective Practice in Nursing*. Blackwell Publishing, Oxford.

reflective writing, whereas reflective writing and critical thinking are the processes, or catalysts, that facilitate these outcomes. Whilst it is convenient to differentiate between these for reasons of clarity, in reality the distinctions between the categories are not so clear-cut, and indeed, they all influence each other in some way.

The solid lines indicate a strong relationship existing between the categories. The broken lines indicate that a weaker relationship appears to exist. Additionally, the arrows linking the concepts are directional. Whilst all the concepts have a relationship with each other and are therefore all essential within the theory, some relationships appear to occur in one direction only.

Activity

Consider Figure 3.2 in relation to your own portfolio.

Does your portfolio contain evidence of these four main elements?

Reflect on the relationships between the categories. How strongly would you say these links relate to you?

Would your portfolio demonstrate your accountability as a practitioner to another person?

Core category: developing evidence of accountable practice

This is the end result of compiling a portfolio that includes reflective writing. The writing component makes the difference between the portfolio being a collection of pieces of paper, such as certificates of attendance, credit or witness statements and other artefacts, and a living document that presents a contemporary picture of the nurse as an accountable professional practitioner. Registration purposes seem to provide the initial stimulation to develop and maintain the portfolio for most nurses. Interestingly, the possibility of litigation which may require them to justify their practice to others, or even in a court of law, seems to be a major reason for committing practice to writing. Although these are major concerns, they are not the primary motivators for writing reflectively, as this comes more from a professional concern to develop practice in order to provide the best possible care for clients.

Accountable practice is perceived as central to professional practice, and is seen as linking the four main categories, with reflective writing being the vehicle for this. Hence, the four main categories have a direct relationship with the notion of accountable practice and, for the nurses, are demonstrated publicly through the process of reflective writing within the portfolio.

Main category one: professional development

The category of documenting and facilitating professional development was initially presented as the main reason for reflective writing. It is comprised of the three subcategories of:

- developing a knowledge base
- evidence of professional practice
- evidence-based practice.

Developing a knowledge base is an essential component of developing professional practice because it is seen as the way that a deeper understanding of practice is developed. This was illustrated by Joe in Case study 3.1.

Moreover, this leads into providing *evidence of professional practice* because that professional practice is based on sound scientific knowledge and working within a professional code of conduct. This results directly in *evidence-based practice* that can be publicly justified. In Joe's case, the team decided not to continue using a herbal remedy that had not been medically prescribed, despite his wife's wishes, because the decision could not be defended with acceptable evidence. In an overt way, the nurses claimed that the reflective components provided evidence of their ongoing development that could be assessed by others, and therefore was visible, or public, in nature.

Hence, there is a strong and direct link between this category and the core category, in that demonstrating professional development is

---

Case study 3.1   Joe's dilemma.

George, a patient with Alzheimer's disease, was admitted to the elderly mental health unit for respite care. His wife, his principal carer, had started using flower remedies to supplement his prescribed medication. Joe, the senior staff nurse, was unhappy about giving medication that was not prescribed, for professional and ethical reasons, but felt torn because the patient's wife clearly felt they were having some effect.

Joe used reflective writing in his portfolio to work through a process of increasing his knowledge base so that he could make informed decisions from the best available evidence. In the end he presented a case to his colleagues justifying a professional decision to refuse to administer the flower remedies. He had done 28 hours research over two days, produced the evidence necessary for the case conference and reflected on the whole incident.

Joe found the process of making the decision very unpleasant, a disagreeable critical incident which he had to justify to himself first of all. He concluded that 'without the process of writing I'd be in trouble, I wouldn't be able to defend the decision'.

---

seen as a key component of demonstrating accountable practice, and reflective writing is perceived as the way that this can be demonstrated.

Summary

- Professional development was identified as the primary stimulus for reflective writing.
- It involves the development of a knowledge base for practice, providing evidence of professional practice and demonstrating evidence-based practice.
- Professional development is seen as fundamental to accountable professional practice.
- It is public in nature.

Main category two: personal development

However, coexistent with professional development is the category of *personal development*, and it appears that these two components exist in a direct and dependent way, in that one will not occur without the other when reflective writing is being used to explore problems and learn from practice. This is significant as it is often assumed that if a person changes then their practice will automatically change as a result. This theory suggests that this is not necessarily the case, as the nurse needs to be aware of the need for change and to take action to effect that change. All the nurses demonstrated, with supporting illustrations, that this had occurred as a result of writing reflectively because the processes enabled them not only to develop a new perspective on a situation, but also to formulate action for it. Thus, the components of the professional development category are not in themselves sufficient to bring about change in behaviour or practice (the simple acquisition of knowledge or evidence will not necessarily result in change). This needs to be accompanied by the attributes of personal development.

Personal development is comprised of four categories:

- reflective writing as a developmental tool
- learning from experience
- cognitive, deliberative process
- developing analytical skills.

Whilst professional development was perceived to be the public, overt representation of themselves within the portfolio, all respondents referred to their development as a person as a result of writing reflectively as a latent, or hidden, outcome. The processes of writing reflectively were viewed as a developmental tool that enables personal insight and growth. Often, acknowledgements of this did not appear in the public portfolio, or if they did, were presented in a sanitised version.

Moreover, the respondents identified private reflective writing as the way they learned from experience. This is interesting, in that the processes that were used were considered to be more rigorous, and more insightful than verbal reflective processes. This is corroborated by evidence from the first stage of the study (Jasper 1999) and illustrated in Case study 3.2.

The fact that the act of writing is a *cognitive, deliberative process* means that it has to be actively engaged in and requires commitment in terms of time, mental and physical energy. It does not occur by accident, but happens consciously and demands cognitive deliberation. The concurrent result is that the nurse is constantly *developing analytical skills*, of which they may or may not be aware. The nurses in this study were, though, very much aware of the effects that using reflective writing were having on them as people and practitioners and felt that they grew as people as a result.

Summary

- Personal development coexists with professional development.
- It occurs as a private part of reflective writing.
- Reflective writing is seen as a developmental tool for personal development.
- Personal development is based on recognising experiential learning through a cognitive, deliberate process.
- This results in the development of analytical skills.

Case study 3.2   Developing self-awareness.

Sue is a senior ward sister tasked with introducing patient-centred care into a unit rife with traditional and routine practices. Her attempts to introduce a new model of practice failed, with consequent feelings of rejection, lack of self-esteem and guilt at the trauma she had caused others. Sue was shocked at the feedback she received from others regarding how she deals with people. She was being perceived as lacking confidence and assertiveness in the way that she had tried to instigate the new methods of working. However, when exploring the issues reflectively she came to realise that the social, cultural and political issues surrounding the change in practice were instrumental in the project's failure. She had almost been set up to fail because she did not receive the support from senior management. She also explored different mechanisms for change management and concluded that a collaborative action research strategy, involving all the staff at the outset, may have been more appropriate than the approach she took. As a result, she developed insight into her inter-professional and communication skills, and developed strategies to develop her confidence in dealing with others. She summarised her feelings in the following way:

'I conclude with the suggestion that my increased self-assurance may be reflected in the ease with which I write in the first person to take ownership of my words.'

Main category three: developing critical thinking

Writing reflectively also impacted on the ways in which the nurses approached the world in terms of the development of critical thinking skills. This is comprised of four subcategories:

- exploring issues
- making connections
- organising thoughts/structures
- taking a new perspective on issues.

These processes were seen as essentially creative, in that they involved unique combinations of *exploring issues* within the elements of the previous knowledge and experience of the practitioner. *Making connections* between previously unrelated and disparate sets of information was seen as a product of reflective writing. One nurse recognised his own creativity with an element of awe; he had developed reflective writing skills as a result of course attendance, and found that it was the mechanism he had been searching for in order to create meaning from his experiences. He was thoroughly committed to the processes, and his writing had become a means of stress relief for him, as well as a mechanism for self-directed learning.

All nurses used the discipline of writing within a reflective structure, be this a recognised one or of their own creation, as a way of *ordering their thoughts/structures.* For some it was important to use a ready-made structure for writing, such as that proposed by Gibbs (1988) or Johns (2002). For others, although they may have initially utilised a pre-given format, it was important to have the flexibility to create a structure appropriate for the topic on which they were reflecting, as differing issues warranted alternative exploratory processes, be this knowledge development, emotional coping strategies or something else. As Ellie (one of the nurses in Jasper's study) said:

> *'It allows you to look at what you have written and to order your thoughts. There is something . . . not just comforting . . . it clarifies your thoughts, just sort of writing everything down. It allows you to take a step back and think, well, maybe this situation isn't as bad as I thought, or, yes it really was not a good situation and I have got to deal with it in some way. It puts everything into perspective and clarifies situations and it is like counselling to some extent in that when you talk through a problem you can stand back from it and think, no, it wasn't as bad as I thought it was. It allows you to prioritise and think 'this is what I do first; from this I do so-and-so . . . It gives you a plan of action.'*

However, the success of using reflective writing appears to be dependent upon the commitment of the person using it. It must be remembered that all the nurses in this study had chosen to use the technique, and therefore had an affinity with it. As a result, the nurses could use reflective writing to work through painful experiences, yet, learn from these in a positive way by putting together the pieces of the experience in a new and creative way.

Summary

- Nurses were aware of the effect of reflective writing on their developing analytical abilities.
- Reflective writing, as a process in its own right, helped them to make connections between ideas, explore issues in different ways, and develop structure and organisation to their thoughts.
- This resulted in taking a new perspective on an experience.

Main category four: outcomes for (clinical) practice

These nurses wanted to be the very best practitioners that they could be. They wanted to demonstrate to the world, in a visible form, that they were affecting patient (or student) outcomes by their practice. In this way they *moved care forward* and delivered the *best patient (or student) care.*

Nurses are clearly learning about, and informing, their professional practice as a result of writing reflectively. This may be stimulated initially by the need to compile a portfolio for registration purposes, but

---

Case study 3.3   Developing a better service.

Mary used her portfolio to back up what she had done in practice. As part of her role as an occupational health nursing sister she set up a blood-taking service within the department. She explored improvement required, the role for her, the implications of it and the course of action needed in her portfolio. She identified that she needed to learn how to take blood, which she did, and was given a certificate to prove her competence. She did some reflective writing six months after setting up the service, asking things like:

Do I feel it is worthwhile?
How has it benefited the service?
Has it enhanced our profile within the hospital?

The results of her personal reflections were then verified with others. The recipients of the service very much appreciated a 'one-stop shop' to enable them to have a consultation and have blood samples taken at the same time instead of having to make another appointment in another part of the hospital. They also appreciated the confidentiality of the service, and not having to wait for attention in the phlebotomy waiting room where they might encounter inquisitive colleagues. Similarly, she went to see the senior phlebotomist and asked whether the occupational health team taking over the service had helped her in any way. Mary received a written reply with a verification to say that, yes, she feels it very much has.

---

it soon becomes an end in itself as one way in which nurses learn experientially. This is illustrated in Case study 3.3.

The results of this study clearly demonstrate the links between reflective writing and professional development, in that the process of writing enables the nurse to develop their critical and analytical abilities, whilst learning experientially from practice. Reflective writing appears to be a catalytic process that results in both professional and personal development by helping the writer to link, and trawl, previously unconnected pieces of information in a creative and innovative way. This ultimately informs practice, and thus facilitates further professional development. The core category of 'developing evidence of accountable practice' draws these together as the *raison d'être* for reflective writing within the portfolio, in that the nurses are proud of their practice, and want to be able to demonstrate their skills as professional practitioners to the outside world.

Summary

- Reflective writing helps to facilitate professional development by providing a dynamic process of critical and analytical thinking to enable the practitioner to learn from their experiences.

- It is the *processes* of reflective writing that results in professional development by creating a unique environment for exploring experience.
- Reflective writing enables the experienced nurse to provide evidence of their accountability as professional practitioners.

Chapter summary

This chapter has reviewed the nature of reflective writing as a strategy for professional development by introducing ways that it can be used within an individual nurse's practice as a professional practitioner. The main message from the chapter is that, to be effective, reflective writing needs to be incorporated within everyday practice, not seen as an adjunct to it. To this end, techniques for using writing have been suggested, and a model of experienced nurses' use of reflective writing within professional portfolios has been presented.

References

Bolton, G. (2005) *Reflective Practice, Writing and Professional Development* (2nd edn). Sage, London.

Bulman, C. and Schutz, S. (ed.) (2004) *Reflective Practice in Nursing* (3rd edn). Blackwell Publishing, Oxford.

Gibbs, G. (1988) *Learning by Doing. A Guide to Teaching and Learning Methods*. Further Education Unit, Oxford Polytechnic, Oxford.

Jasper, M. (1999) Nurses' perceptions of the value of written reflection – the genesis of grounded theory study. *Nurse Education Today*, **19**, 452–463.

Jasper, M. (2003) *Beginning Reflective Practice*. Nelson Thornes, Cheltenham.

Jasper, M. (2004) Learning journals and diary keeping. Chapter five. In: Bulman, C. and Schutz, S. (2004) *Reflective Practice in Nursing* (3rd edn). Blackwell Publishing, Oxford.

Jasper, M. (2006) Developing evidence of accountability: experienced nurses' use of reflective writing in professional portfolios – a grounded theory. Submitted for publication, enquiries to the author.

Jeffrey, A. (2006) *Fast, Focused, Frequent Reflection for Foundation Doctors: a Practical Tool for Learning*. Presentation at the 'Demonstrating competence through reflective writing' conference, 2 February 2006, National Motorcycle Museum, Birmingham.

Johns, C. (2002) *Guided Reflection, Advancing Practice*. Blackwell Publishing, Oxford.

Nursing and Midwifery Council (2004a) *The PREP Handbook*. NMC, London.

Nursing and Midwifery Council (2004b) *Code of Professional Conduct: Standards for Performance, Conduct and Ethics*. NMC, London.

Nursing and Midwifery Council (2005) *Guidelines for Records and Record-keeping*. NMC, London.

Rolfe, G., Freshwater, D. and Jasper, M. (2001) *Critical Reflection for Nursing and the Helping Professions: a User's Guide*. Palgrave, Basingstoke.

Schön, D. (1983) *The Reflective Practitioner*. Temple Smith, London. www. reflectivepractices.co.uk

Decision-making in professional practice

Georgina Koubel

- developed an appreciation of the use of reflective practice in the process of decision-making
- considered the relationship between autonomy, accountability and ethical perspectives in the process of professional decision-making.

Making decisions

Making decisions is something we do every day of our lives. We make decisions for ourselves and for other people. We may make mistakes, take risks and even decide to do something which is not particularly in our own best interests, or even the best interests of others. Using judgement of the context and circumstances that prevail and deciding on a particular course of action is not something that is limited to the workplace. The situation of professionals making decisions within the workplace is nevertheless treated as if it were a completely different matter from the everyday experience of assessment and decision-making that we all carry out within our lives.

Decision-making in everyday life: intuitive and analytical thinking

Decision-making in everyday life requires a number of skills and approaches. Some things, like getting up and washing, we have done so many times that we can do them automatically, almost without thinking. Dressing involves a little more cognition. Although the actual process of getting dressed (outer clothing over underwear, shoes over socks) does not require conscious effort, there are a number of issues that have to be factored into the equation every day, such as the state of the weather, what the wearer will be doing on that day, whether they are taking the car or the bus to work, what's available on the day and what's in the wash, what goes with what, what feels comfortable and what we want to look like to the people we will be seeing on that day. All of these features, whether emotional, or practical, have to be considered when making the apparently simple choice of what to wear.

Then there are the unexpected factors which disrupt the semi-automatic progress of the morning: the childminder rings up sick, or the car won't start. By this time the autopilot is of little use, and we are consciously weighing up the options and choices available to try to decide the best course of action.

It is therefore clear that we are using different methods or frameworks for thinking about different things. Hammond (1983, cited on pp. 81–82 of Dowie and Elstein 1997) identifies a model for clinical decision-making that recognises this process and polarises the ideas of *intuitive* and *analytical* approaches. He suggests that intuitive thinking may be characterised as: 'rapid, unconscious data processing that combines the available information by "averaging" it, it has low consistency and is moderately accurate.' Analytical thought, on the other hand, is: 'slow, conscious and consistent, and is usually quite accurate . . . often combining information using organising principles that are more complicated than simple "averaging".'

Personal and professional decision-making

It appears that the everyday approach to problem-solving requires us to switch between each of these different modes of operating and apply whichever is more appropriate. This indicates that we as human beings have the capacity to operate on a number of different levels and utilise whichever mode is most appropriate for the situation in which we find ourselves. Even so, decision-making at this level does not come under the same scrutiny as that expected from the professional. As Sheppard (1995 p. 7) suggests:

'Faith in the expert knowledge of a profession is crucial to its public acceptance. Such acceptance is dependent on a focus on areas of life believed to be of considerable importance, the possession of skills and knowledge which are difficult to understand and a capacity to bring under control areas of life which would otherwise be plagued by uncertainty. Medicine achieves all these qualities.'

Activity: personal and professional decision-making

Consider the following example:

A neighbour who is visiting you as a friend tells you that she has left her nine-year-old daughter at home on her own because the child has a nasty cough and a slight rash and she wonders whether you can advise what to do about it.

As a *neighbour*, what do you see as your role in this scenario? Would you provide advice? Would you feel it within your remit to examine the child? Would you feel you should address issues of your neighbour leaving a young child alone at home?

If she brought the child into the surgery where you work as a *nurse*, would your response be any different?

In either situation, what would you be basing your judgements and decisions on?

What you need to be thinking about here is the difference between the advice you would feel able to give to someone as a friend, and the difference it would make if you were being consulted in your professional capacity. If you are aware that you would react differently in each of these scenarios, why do you think this is so? Would you be thinking more intuitively or analytically? What issues and concerns would be affecting your judgement in either situation? Can you identify as a nurse what factors would particularly be informing your responses?

Summary

- We all make decisions every day of our lives, from the mundane and the simple to those which are complex and difficult.
- Some decisions are 'intuitive', based on repeated experiences and habits which we have integrated into a set range of knowledge that we can access more or less at will, without even being aware of it. This is not to say that these are not learned activities, but they are so familiar that we no longer need to access the entire learning process to know, for example, how to cross the road.
- Others are 'analytical' and require us to engage consciously and use deliberative cognitive engagement to reach the point of resolution that can be construed as our decision.
- Professional judgement and decision-making have an additional element, in that the decisions made may be open to scrutiny by a range of people, including patients, colleagues, other professional staff, or the public.
- Professional judgement and decision-making may also be measured against legal and ethical frameworks that would not inform our private thoughts and decisions.
- Professional decisions may have to be *accounted for*. Analytical processes can be followed, delineated and demonstrated to others, if necessary. Intuitive actions may be difficult to explain, even when they lead to beneficial outcomes.
- In making decisions as a professional, whether based on intuitive practice wisdom or on critically conscious analysis, you will need to be aware of the possibility that your actions and decisions may be judged against external criteria such as legal and procedural guidelines, targets and standards.

The legal and social context of health care

The current context of health care recognises the complexity of health as part of public and social life. Rapid changes have occurred within the NHS over the past few years and the pace has increased since the return to power of the Labour Party in 1997 (Smith in Chilton *et al.* 2004). There is a strong emphasis on the role of the individual in promoting their own health and well-being but also an awareness of the role of social inequality in the experience of health for different members of society.

The modernisation of health care has led to new developments in the construction of the roles of patient and practitioner, with an avowed intent to recognise health inequalities and provide patients with more information to empower and enable them. However, there are inherent conflicts within the new systems that sometimes make it more difficult to be clear about the role and responsibilities of those involved. Issues of health inequalities are acknowledged in policy but often lie outside the scope of practice. Baggott (2004) suggests that:

'Building on the Major Government's Health of the Nation policy, the Blair Government sought to extend public health beyond efforts to cajole individuals to improve their own lifestyles. [However,] public health strategy continues to be disease focused, emphasising reductions in mortality from the major killers.'

The transformation of patients into customers or consumers of health services has changed the context of health and social care but not in a simple way (Beattie 1992). At the same time, as patients are being expected to become more active and informed about their own condition, medical practitioners appear to have control over resources and therapies that could be withheld from them, with life-affecting consequences for individuals. Expectations are raised by media accounts of the development of new technologies and therapies but decisions about resources remain in the hands of the medical establishment.

This informs individuals about what they, as consumers, should be able to get from their health services, but it is apparent that these treatments are not available on an equal basis to all citizens. In many cases, patients who can afford to do so will chose private options while those who do not have the financial resources may be denied treatment they know to be available. This clearly affects the relationship between patients and practitioners.

Although Sheppard (1995) identifies the level of trust and responsibility granted to professionals within their area of expertise, this is not an area that practitioners can take for granted. Historically, the public has put its faith in the knowledge, skills and perspective of the professional expert, an exchange which allowed people to avoid some of the more difficult and complex decisions around health and death, in return for the power and influence bestowed on professionals. With the emergence of recent scandals, such as those of Dr Harold Shipman and the Alder Hey Hospital, the trust that patients had traditionally accorded medical staff has been brought into question.

In addition, the encouragement by the Government for people to take more responsibility for their own well-being, as well as easy access to the Internet, has enabled patients to develop greater knowledge about their own illnesses and available treatments.

Despite policy documents such as *Building the Best: Choice, Responsiveness and Equity* (Department of Health 2003) which trumpet the value of consultation, decisions about who should receive scarce resources are not automatically accepted by the public, even where there are clear medical indications that, for example, a particular course of treatment will be more beneficial for some people than others.

Shakespeare (2006) argues that this refusal to accept the limits of medical intervention is partly because of the unrealistic expectations that society has of what medicine can and cannot achieve. If people are expected to take greater responsibility for their own health, they are likely to want more say in how resources are allocated and what they feel they should be entitled to from their health service.

A good example of the status of health care in the modern environment is the interest shown regarding the breast cancer drug Herceptin, which was developed as a treatment for the later stages of an aggressive form of breast cancer. Ann Marie Rogers, who had this form of the illness, appealed against the decision of her local primary health care trust not to pay for the drug at the earlier stage of the illness. Although evidence was available that the drug could be effective at an earlier stage, the National Institute of Clinical Excellence (NICE) had not agreed that it *must* be prescribed at the early stage, but some health authorities and trusts were doing so.

The Law Lords acknowledged the problem of the 'postcode lottery' that could arise from local health bodies determining the balance between needs and resources, but did not feel it was their role to tell them what to do. Joan Smith, in the *Independent on Sunday* (19 February 2006 p. 35), however, took issue with this construction of the Modern Agenda in Health Care.

> *'All Ms Rogers is doing is following health managers' advice to take more responsibility for our own health . . . Ms Rogers has taken this to its logical conclusion, doing her homework and concluding quite reasonably that Herceptin might save her life.'*

As Dowie and Elstein (1997) identify, the role of the professional is being held up to scrutiny as never before. The perception of professional expertise is being affected by the changing construction of that role by those both inside and outside the profession, reflected in the requirement for 'greater accountability for professional judgements and decisions.'

Many would welcome the move towards a more equitable distribution of power between practitioners and those patients and clients who have often felt themselves to be at the mercy of professional 'experts' who they feel do not really understand their situation (Shakespeare 2001), or who feel they are better placed to make decisions affecting a person's life than the individual themselves. However, there is a risk that the professional values and standards of the practitioner may conflict with economic and political drivers which affect the scope and range of professional practice in medicine.

Despite the reconstruction of the role of the patient/customer, decisions around the allocation of resources remain with the health bodies, whether at national or local level. However, with increased knowledge and expectations of patients/customers, demand is likely to rise and conflicts are increasingly aired in the public context of legal judgements and, through the media, within the public domain.

While nurses may not have the responsibility to make difficult decisions about who should be eligible to receive drugs such as Herceptin, you may well be the practitioner to whom that person, who has just been refused a drug which they believe could improve or even save their life, will turn. This may involve you in some conflict between the support needs of the patient and your role as an employee of the organisation which has made that decision. Such conflicts are an inevitable part of the role of the nurse working in the changing health care environment, where, as Sir Liam Donaldson (2003) proposes, these developments inevitably change the relationships between patients and practitioners, particularly in the reconstruction of the role of patient as customer or consumer.

> 'Increasingly, people who are being treated by health service agencies legitimately see themselves as customers of that service – a service which they pay for through their taxes. They may make comparisons with other services which they pay for directly. They have expectations as consumers so that part of giving patients respect is also to treat them as they would want to be treated themselves.'

Summary

- Patients are expected to act as consumers and to be part of decision-making in health care.
- Professional practitioners have control and responsibility for the distribution of health care resources.
- Access to health care resources is not equal.
- Professionals, formerly the guardians of knowledge, are increasingly being challenged by the volume of evidence and knowledge available in the public domain.

Values and the ethical context of professional practice

It may be said that professional expertise and the reliance of patients on that expertise is being supplemented if not supplanted by the National Service Frameworks, occupational standards and codes of practice that have been introduced as part of the modernisation agenda for health and social care (Adams 2003 p. 48).

It is within this complex and uncertain environment that nurses must look for the strategies and guidance to enable them to carry out their work in a way that supports and enables patients but which does not place the nurse herself at risk from legal or ethical transgressions. Models of decision-making can help to provide underlying justification for the decisions that practitioners take, but these need to take place within a context of clear communication and transparency. As Walsh (1997 p. 23) puts it:

> *'Accountability means the nurse being able to give an explanation or justification for his or her actions. Practising in this way requires a sound knowledge base upon which to make decisions in conjunction with professional judgement. This decision-making must be transparent, logical and replicable.'*

This suggests that professional decision-making builds upon both *intuitive* and *analytical* processes to incorporate an element of judgement derived from working within professional boundaries and guidelines. To some extent, this supports the notion of 'safe practice' as the practitioner is constantly aware of the repercussions and accountability that underpin their decisions.

The question of logical and replicable decision-making raises a range of issues about the possibility of making logical decisions based on the emotional and traumatic process of working with people who are ill, fearful and often either wishing to ignore the limits and boundaries that medical changes have made in their lives, or who would gladly assign medical practitioners the right to make decisions on their behalf that are not really the remit of those practitioners. Within these areas of uncertainty, it is often the values of the practitioner and the context of anti-oppressive practice that inform the decision-making process (Braye and Preston-Shoot 1994 p. 53).

Activity: professional judgement and personal values

Consider the example of Mrs Betteridge, an 83-year-old widow who lives alone. Admitted to hospital after a fall, she was found to be very dirty, dehydrated and malnourished. Although she is now medically well enough to go home, she

Continued

is still very frail and depends a lot on the nurses for help with personal care activities. Her family, who live some miles away, are very concerned that she will not be able to look after herself and inform you that she will be at risk if she is allowed to go home and live on her own. Mrs Betteridge says she wants to go home but that she doesn't want to upset her family. You are aware of how much better she looks and appears to feel after a period of being looked after in hospital and share some of the family's concerns for how Mrs Betteridge will manage once she is home on her own. She asks you what you think she should do.

How can you help Mrs Betteridge?
What do you think she should do?
As a nurse, what do you feel your role is in this situation?
What advice can you offer?
What are you basing this on?
How comfortable do you feel with this role?

There are a number of views and values that could inform your responses to this or other situations and that could interfere with objectivity and decision-making. No one can be expected to be immune to the culture and society in which they were brought up. It is not possible to avoid any situations in your work which raise ethical issues. In some cases there are specific exemptions, for example in the case of working with women seeking termination of pregnancy, where nurses are expected to declare if they would find this too much of a challenge to their personal beliefs and values.

Other areas which may affect your professional judgement could include racial prejudice, expectations of the role of women or older people, or families who do not appear to provide the care you would expect for their relatives. Like everyone in society, you may have opinions about people who misuse drugs or alcohol, or you may hold particular attitudes in relation to what you think are the needs of people who are disabled, or you may have views about homosexuals or criminals, or you may simply find it difficult to understand people who hold very different values or attitudes to your own. There may even be people who you simply dislike.

At times there may be a conflict between your own values about what you think, personally, would be best for someone and what you can or indeed should do as a nurse. However, it is worth considering whether your own views are affected by ageism or paternalism, whether your good intentions are affected by the need to overprotect or avoid risk on behalf of older people, or to make decisions for people who appear to be vulnerable. Society often takes on a role with older people and people with disabilities that can construe them as needy and dependent, and nurses and indeed older or disabled people themselves are not immune to these models of age or disability (Shakespeare 2001).

Issues of personal choice and autonomy may override what you or others think would be best for individuals who need health and social services, and who can, through their own sense of being powerless and not wanting to upset family members, as in this case, be persuaded to give up their independence even when this is not really what they want to do. Whatever you feel personally about your wish to see her in a safe environment, your role in this situation may be to help Mrs Betteridge achieve what she wants, even acting as an advocate on her behalf to support her wish to live independently if that is what she wants.

This indicates that nurses, and indeed all professional practitioners, have a responsibility to identify and recognise their own views and values and to develop strategies to help them ensure that these do not interfere with decisions that need to be made objectively, based on the evidence available. As Caulfield (2005 p. 32) suggests: 'personal values held by individual nurses are often subsumed by the need to be professional at all times as a nurse.'

Summary

- Everyone is affected and influenced by a range of values, beliefs and attitudes that we develop as we grow up. These may come from family, friends, religion or professional perspectives.
- For professionals who have the power to make decisions that can impact on the lives and well-being of patients, there is a particular responsibility to be aware of the factors which may affect your objectivity and find ways to ensure that your own values and possible prejudices do not intrude on the professional process.

Decision-making models

Theories of decision-making in medicine tend to favour logical, precise, analytical models which are held to be testable, unambiguous and repeatable, therefore satisfying scientific principles. These represent important ideas of certainty and rationality that are intended to provide a sense of security and reliability. Donald Schön (1983), on the other hand, argues that experienced practitioners use a range of strategies, some of which are more intuitive than analytical and which, although based on integrated and accumulated practice wisdom, may actually be difficult to locate within the model of technical rationality. Schön links expertise and high-quality decision-making with concepts of intuition and reflection, both reflection in action and reflection on action, particularly in areas of complexity and uncertainty, which inform and improve the process of professional judgement, intervention and decision-making.

Dowie and Elstein (1997) offer a useful introduction to different models of clinical decision-making which incorporate the spectrum of views linking professional thought and action.

The debate about the theoretical basis of decision-making can lead to polarisation, with intuition or analysis being seen as either a higher or lower form of professional judgement. Hamm (1984), explaining the model of Herbert and Stuart Dreyfus, finds that they maintain that there is a 'fundamental dichotomy' between intuition and analytical thinking.

Dreyfus and Dreyfus argue that different modes, with intuition or analysis, are more relevant to different tasks. Different levels of expertise may also be appropriate for determining which approach is more suitable.

Activity: analysis and intuition

Try to consider these different elements of your role and think how you would approach each of them. Which method would be most appropriate for the following two scenarios: an analytical, evidence-based technical approach, or one which relies on personal experience, practice wisdom or intuition?

(1) making a bed
(2) changing a dressing

What do you see as being the similarities and differences in these two situations?
What skills and knowledge would be involved in either case?
Caulfield (2005) suggests that both of these would involve an intuitive approach. Do you agree?
If not, on what basis would you argue that they are different?

Both of these activities may be so familiar to you that you can complete them without reference to a guide or manual so that they may feel 'intuitive', in that without conscious consideration you can access the best way to carry out each of these activities. Despite this, you will at some stage have learned, either through working with others, or through reading the evidence available around this activity, the best way of undertaking this procedure. You may have incorporated the process into your practice wisdom so thoroughly that you can carry out both of these procedures almost without being aware of the steps involved.

This does not mean that they are both the same. One key factor that should alert you to the difference depends on the involvement of the patient as person or individual. While the bed cannot object or agree to the procedure, the patient can. They may be distressed, scared, in pain, aggressive, resistant or grateful for your help. The *National Service Framework for Older People* (Department of Health 2002) emphasises at every stage the importance of *person-centred care*.

You need, therefore, to think about how your intervention can encompass the values and skills involved in person-centred care, and whether this utilises the skills of intuition or analysis. You also need to be aware that in all your activities you are employing some models of working. Once the judgements or decisions become more complex, it is to these models that you can turn for help in resolving difficulties.

Models such as Hammond's Cognitive Continuum posit the concept of six levels of judgement: intuitive, peer-aided, system-aided, epidemiological study, controlled trial and scientific experiment (Dowie and Elstein 1997). The idea that both the complexity of the task and the level of expertise of the practitioner will influence the method of decision-making and professional judgement recognises the difficulty of allocating a specific model to a particular circumstance. In reality, the process is negotiated taking into account a range of issues which will influence the way in which these processes are managed.

Decision analysis, which has been widely employed in medical care, tries to reconcile the rights and perspectives of the individual with the need of the system to target the most effective use of valuable medical resources. By assigning numerical or 'objective' properties to utilities or medical options and personal preferences or 'values' this model attempts to determine preferential outcomes in cases of difficulty or complexity. It is hoped that this will somehow satisfy the needs of the individual patient while providing a rational and logical account of the reasons underpinning that decision.

Sometimes this may be done in relation to a particular person's circumstances, while at others it may inform national or local policy. An example of this may be decisions not to provide new kidneys for people with drink problems, or to refuse hip operations to people who are obese. While objectively these treatments may be better targeted towards those who do not have such qualities, how ethical is it to deny treatments that could relieve pain and suffering, or even maintain life, to people because of their lifestyle? Issues of quality of life and personal preference are not always subject to the clarity of objective reasoning. As Bruner (1987 p. 13) says: 'There is heartlessness about logic.'

Summary

- Theories of decision-making in medicine favour logical, precise, analytical models which are held to be testable, unambiguous and repeatable, therefore satisfying scientific principles.

- Professional practitioners supplement this technical-rational model with intuition and reflection on experience – clinical expertise.
- Different models of decision-making are appropriate for different tasks.

A process model of decision-making – using the 5WH cues

Taking into account the balance between the intuitive and analytical approaches to professional judgement and decision-making, there is a strong argument for a model that enables practitioners to take into account the emotional, ethical elements of person-centred practice while retaining a level of objectivity which incorporates valid reference to research and evidence. This model of decision-making relies on the practitioner asking a range of relevant questions:

- what?
- why?
- who?
- when?
- where?
- how?

Using this *process model of decision-making*, the practitioner needs to be aware of *what* the problem is, *why* it is a problem (and why it is a problem *now*), *who* it is a problem *for*, *when* and *where* it is a problem, and *how* the people involved can find the best methods or strategies to deal with the problem.

Issues of perspectives and priorities are important here, as different people (or stakeholders) who have an interest in resolving the problem may have different opinions both about what the problem is, and the best ways of dealing with it.

Perry and Parsons (cited in Chilton *et al.* 2004) identify some of the major factors which need to be considered by practitioners, particularly in the community. These include:

- the local agenda
- the client agenda
- the professional agenda
- the Government agenda
- resources
- partnership working.

The following example can help you think about the benefits of using this model of decision-making.

Activity: the process model of decision-making

Jakob Lesnovic is a Hungarian man of 55 who has lived in the UK for the past 12 years, and who has been diagnosed with schizophrenia. He has recently moved to a small rented flat in an area which has a mixture of private and rented accommodation. Despite his medication, Jakob sometimes becomes quite disturbed and restless, particularly at night, often making a noise and waking other residents, some of whom are elderly and some of whom have young children. The neighbours have approached you to ask whether Jakob could be rehoused in a different neighbourhood, but Jakob says he feels settled in his flat, and says that without the support he gets from fellow Hungarian émigrés who live fairly nearby, his mental health problems would be much worse. Taking a process model of decision-making, you need to think about:

What is the problem? Is it Jakob's mental health or is it the fact that he is disturbing his neighbours?
Who is it a problem for? What are the conflicts between the needs and rights of Jakob and those of his neighbours?
Where and when is it a problem?
How can it be addressed? Is there any research, evidence or practice wisdom that you can access to negotiate the best possible resolution of this situation?

The above provides a good example of a situation where, as a nurse working in the community, you will have professional concern for the medical needs and human rights of your patient but may also sympathise with the genuine concerns that the neighbours are asking you to address. To this scenario, you bring specific knowledge and expertise which can help you think about each stage of the decisions you need to make in this case.

For example, you should be aware that under the Mental Health Act 1983 you, and other professionals from psychiatry and social work, would need to be convinced that Jakob was a danger to himself or others before you could remove him compulsorily from his home. Article 5 (the right to liberty and security of the person) of the Human Rights Act 1998 could also be relevant in protecting Jakob's entitlement to stay in his present accommodation (www.dh.gov.uk/ PolicyAndGuidance/EqualityAndHumanRights2006).

Other considerations, such as the values and possible prejudices of the neighbours around Jakob's nationality or their fears about the impact of his mental health problems, may be significant, in which case some 'educative' elements may be helpful in explaining to the neighbours the limitations of your legal role and then perhaps advocating on Jakob's behalf by reassuring them about the potential risks that they fear Jakob may pose. It may also be helpful for you to make sure Jakob is aware of the worries his neighbours have, and help him appreciate that they need a reasonable expectation of peace and quiet at night. Equally, there may be other issues for Jakob relating to medication or possible alcohol or substance misuse that could be addressed, which could help to reduce the disturbance posed by Jakob in the night-time when other residents are trying to sleep. Rather than taking a purely 'scientific' or 'medical' approach to the problem, a process model of decision-making could help to meet the needs of the various parties involved and improve the situation for everyone by reducing the conflict between Jakob and his neighbours.

Summary

- A balanced approach to decision-making needs to be taken between rational and intuitive models.
- This can be represented as a process model.
- This approach enables a range of factors to be considered that are pertinent to the individual.
- Factors external to the individual, such as Government legislation and local policies, will also be part of this process.

Decision-making in practice

According to Perry and Parsons (cited in Chilton *et al.* 2004), the current context of nursing practice requires a range of skills which may include the following, depending on whether the nurse is working in hospital or in the community:

- the assessment of individuals and families
- decision-making
- clinical expertise
- health promotion
- teaching
- understanding and respect for the client, culture and community
- effective communication skills, underpinning all of the above.

Decisions are not made in isolation from the context in which they are made, and will be influenced by the Government agenda, the client or patient's agenda (which may or may not be the same as their family or carer's agenda), the nurse's (and very likely other disciplines') professional agenda, the current context of health care, including issues of choice, responsibility, partnership and resources. Within this multifaceted arena, nurses need to find strategies for dealing with the complexities of practice.

In the Nursing and Midwifery Council's (2004) *Code of Professional Conduct*, a range of professional and ethical issues are addressed, including the need for practitioners:

- to respect the patient as an individual
- to obtain consent before the implementation of any treatment or care
- to cooperate with others in the team
- to protect confidential information
- to act to identify and minimise risk to patients.

These establish the ethical and values framework within which a nurse is expected to practise. On top of these will be a range of policies and procedures, as well as standards of behaviour expected by Government, your employer and your patients.

It is important to be aware of the processes, guidelines and protocols that we draw on when making decisions and professional judgements. In looking at models of decision-making and the factors that influence professional judgement, it becomes apparent that, particularly in more complex situations, we depend on a wide range of elements. These would include:

- legal and procedural guidelines
- our own and professional ethics
- codes of conduct
- resources available
- knowledge and skills base
- available evidence of best practice
- experience
- clinical judgement
- the views of other professionals
- the choices and capacity of the patient and his/her carers
- decisions made in similar situations
- reflection on action, that is, reflective practice.

Activity: confidentiality and concern

Decision-making within the realities of professional practice is not always simple and there are times when these requirements may conflict with each other. Try to identify which elements of the *Code of Conduct* are relevant in this scenario:

Mrs Shah is a 29-year-old woman from an Asian background who was recently admitted to hospital to have her third baby. There were a number of complications and in the time she has been in hospital you have been quite friendly towards her. Her English is not good but you seem able to understand her. You have seen her husband visiting Mrs Shah and have observed that his manner towards her is very brusque and often when he leaves Mrs Shah looks

Continued

upset. When you go to see her about discharge arrangements, she bursts into tears and says she doesn't know how she will manage. You ask her about her husband, but although she admits he can be verbally and, on occasion, physically aggressive, Mrs Shah is adamant that she does not want anything done about this. She says that this would bring shame on the family and that she only told you about him because she trusted that you would not tell anyone else.

What decisions do you need to consider in this situation?
What are the legal and ethical issues regarding confidentiality?
Can you identify additional issues relating to cultural awareness that may be relevant?

In the NMC *Code of Professional Conduct* there appears to be a conflict between the need to maintain confidentiality and the need to identify and manage risk to the patient. By alerting the authorities to your concerns, you would appear to be dealing with issues of risk but potentially breaking the code of confidentiality, and possibly breaching the need to respect the autonomy of the individual.

There is an additional factor in this situation, in the cultural aspects of this case. Dobash and Dobash (1998 p. 53) sum up the dilemma that this situation poses for both the patient and the practitioner:

'The woman of colour who lives in a racialist society and is also beaten by her partner faces impossible choices. She may escape her man's violence but at the cost of family and community solidarity or she may remain ensconced within family and community but at the cost of her personal safety and well-being.'

There are a number of ways in which this problem can be addressed. One would be to adhere to the professional duty of confidentiality which requires nurses to maintain the trust patients place in them. There is a legal requirement to maintain confidentiality and the practitioner could be liable legally should the breaching of confidentiality lead to damage to the parties who had a right to expect that their information was given in confidence. Furthermore, the 'duty of trust is at the heart of the concept of confidentiality' (Caulfield 2005 p. 142).

The decision to maintain confidentiality in this instance may also be based on the ethical grounds of Mrs Shah's autonomy and respect for her choices, which is a prime consideration within the NMC *Code of Professional Conduct*. However, this may conflict with other ethical imperatives around duty of care and doing what is in the best interests of the patient.

In this scenario, the practitioner may fear that by pursuing the issue there is a risk that a potentially volatile situation could be exacerbated.

However, this leaves the nurse with concerns for Mrs Shah's well-being, and raises the spectre of other (possible) risks to the children, including the possibility of risk to the newborn baby who, it could be argued, is also a patient. The baby would clearly need to be protected from harm as an infant with no capacity to protect himself, but at this stage there is no direct evidence to even indicate that harm to the child is a possibility.

On the other hand, it could be argued that this is not a medical problem but one which has social implications. However, this does not simplify the matter. By highlighting the risk of violence to Mrs Shah, and possibly encouraging her to take action to protect herself, the practitioner may be exposing Mrs Shah to rejection by the family, culture and community that may form her main sources of support and possibly the best chance she has to gain help and protection. By not confronting the issues, the practitioner could be accused of colluding with issues of risk and concern.

The conflict appears to hinge on the duty to respect confidentiality against the nurse's duty of care, which in part may be met by respecting confidentiality (Dimond 2002). In the case of a child, there may well be circumstances where confidences would have to be disclosed to the appropriate people. With vulnerable adults, there is equally a requirement to pass on information if not to do so would leave the person at risk.

In the case of Mrs Shah, your judgement about her level of vulnerability is not laid down by law; as an autonomous person she has a right to have her confidentiality respected. However, if you feel there are sufficient risks to her welfare that you should at least share the information with other members of the multi-professional team, then you should do so. It is then the responsibility of the team to determine their actions, taking account of the concerns relating to confidentiality.

Looking for guidance may also be difficult. Hutchinson and Baker (1999) propose that guidelines for clinical practice can provide 'tools not rules' which can assist practitioners with difficult decisions but cannot make the decisions for them. They do, however, identify the importance of involving patients in the decision-making process, although the level of involvement may be seen as variable. This leaves you once again with the need to balance the expressed wishes of Mrs Shah for you to respect her confidentiality against your concerns about risks to her and her children.

It is likely that your employer will have a set of policies and procedures to assist the practitioner in these kinds of complex problems, but once again the element of professional judgement (about the level of risk, the risk to others) and the consequences of taking action or not will fall to you as the practitioner. One option may be to discuss this with other colleagues in the team. This connects along Hammond's continuum as 'peer-aided' decision-making, which may be part of the culture of the hospital.

Other options involve explaining to the patient the options that are available to her, ensuring she has access to information about the agencies that she may wish to approach, such as housing, social services and Women's Aid, and discussing the use of a Health Visitor who has a role in visiting all newborn babies and may therefore be accepted within the family network as a non-threatening professional who could monitor the children's progress while keeping an eye on Mrs Shah. These may open up the possibilities that Mrs Shah could pursue should she decide at some stage to remove herself from risk, while also ensuring that the children are not being placed at 'significant harm' (Children Act 1989) by being left in the situation.

Other sources of support may come from within the clinical team or from other members of the multi-professional team (Ovretveit *et al.* 2003). Government papers such as *No Secrets* (Department of Health 2001) stress the importance of involving other professionals in the decision-making process to ensure that professionals are communicating and working together effectively to protect vulnerable adults from harm.

One element that is essential for practitioners involved in complex areas such as this would be the recording of relevant information in a way that highlights the concerns but which deals with facts. Often it is not possible to establish a picture of 'the truth' of a given situation but it is important that any reports are based as far as possible on the evidence actually seen by the practitioner or using the actual words of the individual. Where impressions or unsubstantiated areas of concern do need to be recorded, it is vital that the report makes clear where opinions are being expressed.

The decision to keep a record or to pass information to social services may be useful. Even where the decision is to take no action this would at least have the benefit of highlighting the issues in this family in case of future concerns arising, and would also provide an audit of accountability for the decisions made.

In such situations of complexity and uncertainty, there is some value in considering the balance of risk and autonomy, and in some cases a numerical model may be useful in assessing the level of risk (Kent County Council Risk Assessment 2002). However, in view of the difficulty of providing a numerical value when so much is unknown about the situation, strategies such as supervision and reflective practice may provide the most useful route for practitioners to develop their levels of understanding.

It is often the case that nurses are required to respond urgently to a quickly changing situation and frequently their reactions may of necessity be based on previous experience or knowledge. As nurses move into areas of practice which further challenge their traditional roles, such as nurse prescribing, there is evidence that their knowledge and skills remain crucial to the process of professional judgement and decision-making. Jennifer Humphries in Humphries and Green (2002 p. 51) found that:

> 'Research looking at decision-making in the context of nurse prescribing (Luker et al. 1998) . . . noted that while there is a move towards more evidence-based practice, nurses continue to use experiential knowledge, for example previous experience of conditions and knowledge of the patient/client.'

Summary

- Decisions are not made in isolation from the context in which they are made.
- Professional decisions need to be made from inside the values and ethical codes of behaviour established by the Nursing and Midwifery Council and your employer.
- The patient's cultural context also needs to inform decision-making at the individual level.
- An understanding of the nature of confidentiality is central to decision-making.
- Part of the professional's role is to facilitate and support others in making decisions, particularly in relation to the individual patient and decisions about their own care and future care.
- Issues of risk and autonomy need to be considered.
- Knowledge and skill remain at the heart of professional decision-making.

Accountability

One of the most important factors in decision-making is that of accountability. This raises the question of accountability to whom. Caulfield (2005) proposes a model of four pillars of accountability or authority for professional intervention. She identifies the importance of professional, legal and ethical accountability but also recognises the need for nurses to be aware of their accountability to employers in following required policies and procedures. (Accountability is dealt with in more detail in Chapter 8.) Although it is important for practitioners to involve patients in decision-making, nurses also have to face up to the complexity of decision-making in areas which highlight conflicts around capacity and consent. In many cases this may involve practitioners walking the fine line between autonomy and paternalism.

Activity: accountability

Mrs Betteridge, who we met earlier, has asked you to advocate for her with her family to let them know that she definitely wants to pursue her decision to return home. When you talk to the family, they are upset and angry, and insist that it will be your responsibility if she goes home and anything bad happens to her.

How will you respond to this issue of your professional accountability?
Can you list the decision-making tools you use in your practice?
Can you list the assessment tools you use in your practice?
Can you identify how this helps you to promote good practice in decision-making and accountability?

While her family have every right to be concerned about Mrs Betteridge, she has an equal right to make decisions for herself. However, you need to demonstrate the basis for your decision to support her in this. In considering this, you could make reference to:

- national service frameworks
- your *Code of Professional Conduct*
- the medical guidelines, policies and procedures
- legal issues around capacity and human rights
- your assessment of Mrs Betteridge's needs, rights and choices
- your empathy with the personal preferences of the individual while recognising the concerns of those who will be caring for her once she leaves hospital.

Communication is an absolutely vital element of any accountability. As such, you need to think about who needs to know what, ensuring that the format in which any information is provided is accessible to those concerned, and make sure that everyone is clear about who can be contacted if there are any problems or changes in circumstances. Often relatives are afraid to allow someone to take any risks because they fear they will not know what to do if the situation deteriorates, and good communication about support networks can often help to reassure relatives that they will not be left alone when problems arise.

Summary

- Professionals are accountable for the decisions they make.
- Four types of accountability have been identified: professional, legal, ethical and employer.
- Communication is a vital element of accountability.

Capacity and consent

Patient autonomy is usually held to be paramount. Although there is a certain duty of care associated with professional judgement, every human being of adult years and of sound mind has a right to determine what should be done with his/her own body (Dimond 2003). If, however, there are doubts about the mental capacity of that individual to make an informed judgement about what is best for them, this raises concerns for professionals involved with the individual in trying to determine what would be considered to be in their best interests.

Activity: capacity and consent

This example will help to identify the issues that can arise in such circumstances.

Mr Brown is a 75-year-old man who has been known to both health and social services in the past as a carer for his wife who died a few months ago. He now appears rather confused and forgetful at times, but he is often able to hold lucid conversations. Following the death of his wife, Mr Brown was admitted to hospital where investigations revealed that he has stomach cancer. The consultant has said that Mr Brown should have an operation which offers a good chance of recovery but Mr Brown is adamant that he does not want any treatment; he just wants to go home to die. Family members are very upset and ask you to try to persuade Mr Brown to have the operation.

There are a number of questions that could help you to look at what decisions need to be made in this case.

(1) Does Mr Brown have the capacity to make the decision about treatment?
(2) Has he been declared medically or legally incompetent?
(3) If so, can the family make decisions on his behalf?
(4) If he is felt to have capacity, what should your role be in urging Mr Brown to undergo the operation?
(5) What would help you in deciding how to approach this problem?

The situation here appears to rest to a large extent on whether Mr Brown can be said to be legally competent under the Mental Health Act 1983 to make the decision as to whether or not he should have the operation. This would need to be assessed by a psychiatric consultant, preferably one with experience in working with older people. If it is determined that Mr Brown has capacity, no one else can make the decision for him. If not, it would be helpful to know whether he has expressed previously, when he did have capacity, any opinions about whether he would want to undergo surgery in such an event.

It is possible, however, that Mr Brown's reluctance to accept medical treatment may be more to do with his sadness at the loss of his wife than a real reluctance to undergo surgery. He is likely to be undergoing a bereavement process where he is experiencing a sense of loss. This may be resulting in an inability to see the value in prolonging his own life now that he no longer has his life partner to share it with.

This may or may not be affecting his capacity for decision-making, and may require a period of counselling to explore the options that are available to him and put the medical issues into perspective. It is important not to assume that any refusal to give consent to what appears to be a reasonable medical intervention is a sign of incapacity; there may be many other reasons for the individual to make this decision. These may include depression, fear of medical procedures, lack of trust in the medical profession or a reluctance to endure the illness or indignities that may be associated with invasive surgery. You need to consider the significance of the specific reason for this particular individual's refusal to give consent rather than make assumptions about its meaning in general. As Caulfield (2005 p. 137) suggests:

> *'The importance of a refusal (to give consent) from an adult seems to be that it triggers a fresh evaluation of understanding, but it does not mean, because the person refuses to agree with the nurse's proposal, that he or she has necessarily lost the understanding that is crucial to give consent. There have been no cases dealing with this problem which would provide legal guidance.'*

In trying to weigh up the options in this situation, it is important to be aware that it is not acceptable for practitioners to place undue influence in trying to persuade the patient to receive treatment. Your role may entail exploring with the family Mr Brown's rights in respect of refusing treatment. Clearly, there is a responsibility to ensure Mr Brown and the family have all the available information, and in a format that they can understand. Professionals are often unaware of how difficult it is for patients and their families to participate in decision-making, purely because of the opacity of medical language to those who are not familiar with it rather than because they are unable to understand the issues involved if explained clearly.

Summary

- It is important not to assume that because someone refuses medical treatment that other people see as reasonable they are thereby demonstrating that they are incapable of making that decision.
- The decision about capacity can only be determined by a suitably qualified and experienced medical practitioner.
- If the patient does have capacity, you should not use undue influence to persuade the patient to accept any treatment that they do not want.

- It is not clear whether families can legally make decisions on behalf of someone who has limited or fluctuating mental capacity, but any information provided previously regarding their views could be taken into account.
- There is a new but controversial proposal by Government that individuals can nominate a relative or a friend to make such decisions in the case of incapacity.

Chapter summary

The conclusion that nurses' decision-making tends to be based on a range of both analytical and intuitive processes, incorporating both 'theoretical knowledge and knowledge from professional practice experience' (Higgs and Titchen 2001 p. 4) is not surprising. Working across a range of contexts and within areas of increasing complexity, it may at times prove difficult for the practitioner to really explain the reasons for the decisions and actions involved at a particular time. Reflection on action (Schön 1983), after the crisis has passed, can provide an invaluable tool for understanding the reasons behind actions taken and learning new ways of dealing with complexity in the future (Rolfe *et al.* 2001).

There is so much information in the public domain now that there is Governmental expectation that patients and public involvement in decision-making will be at the heart of the modernisation agenda for health (Department of Health 2006). This has led to a situation where medical practitioners have to be aware of both the rights of their patients and the possibility of legal action. However, Caulfield (2005) stresses that in this climate there is a real risk of defensive practice that could lead to routinised, unconsidered or procedure-led practice that does not really meet the needs of patients or fully employ the skills and knowledge of the professionals involved in working with them.

Summary of key points

- There are important differences in decision-making as a professional and as a private person.
- The process of professional judgement involves an awareness of both intuitive and analytical thinking. You need to be aware of when it is important to change from one to the other, or to use both.
- One of the key aspects for nurses is working with people. You should be aware of personal values and ethical frameworks, and the fact that these may conflict. Although person-centred care is an essential component of working with patients and their families, there are other factors, such as the needs of the individual versus

their families, the needs of the institution and commitment to society, and issues of capacity, risk and vulnerability which may impact on the absolute autonomy of the individual or the nurse's unassailable duty of confidentiality.

- Theoretical models can provide useful frameworks but need to be tailored to address the situation, the complexity of the task and the level of experience of the practitioner. A process model of decision-making, as discussed in this chapter, is a useful way of approaching the complexities and realities of decision-making in practice.
- Professional judgement and decision-making is closely allied to issues of accountability. Helen Caulfield's (2005) four pillars of accountability provide a good overview of the elements that need to be addressed in relation to the professional role. Other areas that can inform professional judgement and decision-making include clinical guidance from the Department of Health and the National Institute for Clinical Excellence, alongside information around ethics from the Nursing and Midwifery Council. Government targets and guidance, clinical supervision and institutional procedures may all be relevant.
- Legal issues have to be taken into account, and it is important that you should be aware of the legal frameworks which have relevance for your role and practice. However, it is crucially important not to fall into the trap of routine risk-averse treatment which could ignore the real needs and wishes of the patient.
- Management and supervision processes available for practitioners in practice provide important sources of consultation and support for practitioners facing difficult decisions (Jasper and Jumaa 2005).
- Reflective practice is another invaluable way of improving your professional judgement and decision-making. As well as providing opportunities to review and evaluate effectiveness, reflection helps in the task of maintaining that vital awareness of the patient as a person with feelings, rights and needs which are part of the decision-making process. It also assists in the process of becoming conscious of how your own personal values and prejudices may affect your professional judgement and decision-making in the complex and uncertain context of contemporary professional practice.

References

Adams, A. (2003) *The Modernisation of Social Work Practice and Management in England*. Eichstatt, BK-Verlag Stassfurt, Czech Republic.

Baggott, R. (2004) *Health and Health Care in Britain* (3rd edn). Palgrave, Basingstoke.

Beattie, A. (1992) *Health and Well-being*. Macmillan Educational, Houndsmill.

Braye, S. and Preston-Shoot, M. (1994) *Empowering Practice in Social Care*. Open University Press, Buckingham.

Bruner, J.S. (1987) *Actual Minds, Possible Worlds*. Harvard University Press, London.

Caulfield, H. (2005) *Vital Notes for Nurses: Accountability*. Blackwell Publishing, Oxford.

Chilton, S., Melling, K., Drew, D. and Clarridge, A. (2004) *Nursing in the Community: an Essential Guide to Practice*. Hodder, London.

Department of Health (1983) *Mental Health Act*. Her Majesty's Stationery Office (HMSO), London.

Department of Health (1989) *Children Act*. HMSO, London.

Department of Health (2001) *No Secrets: Guidance on Developing and Implementing Multi-agency Policies and Procedures to Protect Vulnerable Adults from Abuse*. Department of Health, London.

Department of Health (2002) *National Service Framework for Older People*. Department of Health, London.

Department of Health (2003) *Building the Best: Choice, Responsiveness and Equity*. Department of Health, London.

Department of Health (2006) *Our Health, Our Care, Our Say*. Department of Health, London.

Dimond, B. (2002) *Legal Aspects of Patient Confidentiality*. BJN Monographs Quay Books, Wiltshire.

Dimond, B. (2003) *Legal Aspects of Consent*. BJN Monographs Quay Books, Wiltshire

Dobash, R.E. and Dobash, R.P. (1998) *Rethinking Violence Against Women*. Sage Publications, Thousand Oaks, CA.

Donaldson, Sir Liam (2003) Foreword. In: Wright, J. (ed.) *Clinical Governance*. Churchill Livingstone, Edinburgh.

Dowie, J. and Elstein, A. (eds) (1997) *Professional Judgement: a Reader in Clinical Decision-making* (4th edn). Cambridge University Press, Cambridge.

Hamm, R.M. (1984) Clinical intuition and clinical analysis: expertise and the cognitive continuum. In: Dowie, J. and Elstein, A. (eds) (1996) *Professional Judgement: a Reader in Clinical Decision-making*. Cambridge University Press, Cambridge.

Higgs, J. and Titchen, A. (2001) *Practice Knowledge and Expertise in the Health Professions*. Butterworth-Heinemann, Oxford.

Humphries, J.L. and Green, J. (eds) (2002) *Nurse Prescribing* (2nd edn). Palgrave, Hampshire.

Hutchinson, A. and Baker, R. (eds) (1999) *Making Use of Guidelines in Clinical Practice*. Radcliffe Medical Press Ltd, Oxford.

Jasper, M. and Jumaa, M. (eds) (2005) *Effective Health Care Leadership*. Blackwell Publishing, Oxford.

Kent County Council (2002) *Risk Assessment*. KCC, Maidstone.

Nursing and Midwifery Council (2004) *Code of Professional Conduct: Standards for Performance, Conduct and Ethics*. NMC, London.

Ovretveit, J. (2003) *Evaluating Health Interventions*. Open University Press, Maidenhead.

Rolfe, G., Freshwater, D. and Jasper, M. (2001) *Critical Reflection for Nursing and the Helping Professions*. Palgrave Macmillan, Hampshire.

Schön, D.A. (1983) *The Reflective Practitioner*. Basic Books, New York.

Shakespeare, T. (2001) *Help*. Venture Press, Birmingham.

Shakespeare, T. (2006) *The Independent*, 23 January 2006.

Sheppard, M. (1995) *Care Management and the New Social Work*. University of Sheffield, Joint Unit for Social Services Research, Sheffield.

Smith J. (2006) *Independent on Sunday*, 19 February 2006 p. 35.

Walsh, M. (1997) Accountability and intuition: justifying nursing practice. *Nursing Standard*, **11** (23) 26 February, pp. 39–45.

Wright, J. (2003) *Clinical Governance*. Churchill Livingstone, Edinburgh.

Webliography

www.dh.gov.uk/Publications/PublicationsLibrary
Building on the best: choice, responsiveness and equity in the NHS. Accessed 18 January 2006.

www.dh.gov.uk/PolicyAndGuidance/EqualityAndHumanRights
Human rights case studies. Accessed 18 January 2006.

Evidence-based practice

5

Gary Rolfe

Learning objectives

This chapter surveys the literature on evidence-based practice (EBP) from its origins in medicine to the present-day disputes over how it might be applied to nursing. It recognises the controversies surrounding EBP, and attempts to engage critically with the various viewpoints rather than trying to arrive at a consensus which does not actually exist. For this reason, this chapter does not provide any clear-cut answers to questions such as 'What is EBP?' and 'How can I practise in an evidence-based way?' It attempts to *raise* rather than *answer* questions, and to engage readers in their own explorations of the literature, leading them to formulate some answers of their own.

By the end of this chapter, the reader will have:

- an understanding of the significance of the various evidence-based terminology
- critically examined the different types of evidence employed in EBP
- examined different hierarchies of evidence, including similarities and differences between them
- explored different approaches to judging competing forms of evidence, including judgements based on hierarchies and judgements based on expertise
- examined the difficulties involved in making evidence-based decisions
- understood some of the reasons why evidence-based practice remains such a contested concept.

Introduction

There is little doubt that evidence-based practice (EBP) has caught the imagination of the nursing profession during the past decade, and its use is now so widespread and perhaps even taken for granted that it is becoming difficult to find a nurse who would not admit to being an evidence-based practitioner. As Feinstein and Horwitz (1997) observed, it is perhaps difficult to see how anyone could possibly object to the idea of basing practice on best evidence, since the alternatives would be to practise on less-than-best evidence or even on no evidence at all. However, when asked what they understand by EBP, nurses often answer in a variety of different ways. Not only do different practitioners have different views about what precisely should count as *evidence* for practice, they also disagree on which aspects of *practice* should be evidence-based and just exactly what it means to *base* their practice on evidence. We can perhaps begin to see, then, that all three words of the seemingly innocuous phrase 'evidence-based practice' could mean different things to different nurses.

Activity

Before we go any further, perhaps this is a good time to ask yourself what EBP means to you.

The aim of this chapter is to provide you with some of the views offered by eminent writers in the field of nursing and medicine so that you can begin to think a little more about the confusion and controversy surrounding the issue, and come to your own conclusions about the nature of evidence-based practice.

What is evidence-based practice?

Terminology

Perhaps a good starting point for our discussion is with terminology. You will see that this chapter is titled 'evidence-based practice', and yet anyone familiar with the literature will notice that there are several other terms that appear to be used almost interchangeably, including evidence-based nursing, evidence-based medicine and evidence-based health care. French (2002 p. 253) recently charted the number of publications which included these different terms (Table 5.1), from the first recorded use of 'evidence-based medicine' in 1992, through to the year 2000.

Table 5.1   The growth of the concept of evidenced-based practice.

	Evidence-based medicine	Evidence-based practice	Evidence-based nursing
1992	1		
1993	5		
1994	11	1	
1995	69	6	
1996	214	27	1
1997	595	62	13
1998	845	64	8
1999	1464	104	13
2000	1642	110	8

We can see that the use of the term 'evidence-based medicine' (EBM) has grown rapidly, and that 'evidence-based practice' (EBP) was introduced two years after and has also shown an increase in use, although not to the same extent. The term 'evidence-based nursing' (EBN) was first coined in 1996 and does not appear to have caught on in quite the same way.

These differences in terminology are important, and should not be seen simply as different ways of saying the same thing. Whereas 'evidence-based *practice*' is beginning to be used as a way of extending the ideas of evidence-based medicine into other healthcare disciplines such as nursing and midwifery, the term 'evidence-based *nursing*' is usually employed to *distinguish* nursing from medicine. In other words, when nurses use the term EBP they are usually aligning themselves with the EBM movement, whereas when they use the term EBN, they are generally pointing out the differences between nursing and medicine. We can see this distancing of EBN from EBM quite clearly in Mulhall's warning to nurses that: 'tiptoeing in the wake of the movement for evidence-based medicine, however, we must ensure that evidence-based nursing attends to what is important for nursing.' (Mulhall 1998 p. 4)

We can see that whereas Mulhall might accept the basic underlying views of the evidence-based medicine movement, she was very keen to point out that nursing has a somewhat different agenda. Whilst we have adopted the term 'evidence-based practice' in this chapter, we will also be looking at the emerging evidence-based nursing movement.

Activity

Make a few notes on what you mean by 'evidence' or would consider to be evidence that you could use in your practice. I'll ask you to refer back to this after reading the next two sections.

Evidence from research

When you asked yourself what EBP meant to you, I suspect that research figured somewhere in your answer. Whilst almost all nurses agree that research findings play an important role in EBP, there is a surprising lack of consensus about how this research might be evaluated and applied to practice. For some nurses, this might not appear to be a particularly interesting or relevant question, since it is possible for a nurse to practise in an evidence-based way without ever encountering any raw evidence, or indeed, even realising that they are doing evidence-based practice. So, for example, nurses who follow nursing guidelines, NICE (National Institute for Clinical Excellence) recommendations and care pathways are almost certainly basing their practice on research evidence, although they might not be aware of it.

For others, doing evidence-based practice means basing practice wherever possible on the findings of 'gold standard' research studies such as randomised controlled trials (RCTs). This approach to EBP derives directly from medicine, and tends to judge the quality of evidence according to the quantitative research criteria of validity and reliability. David Evans argues that, for nurses: 'ranking research designs according to their internal validity not only grades the strength of the evidence, but also indicates the confidence the end-user can have in the findings' (Evans 2003 p. 78).

Evans proposes that we judge evidence derived from *all* research methodologies, both quantitative and qualitative, as well as evidence from other sources such as expert opinion, according to these quantitative criteria. Furthermore, he argues that these criteria are always the most relevant for judging evidence, regardless of the clinical situation that nurses might find themselves in. Whether they are judging the effectiveness of a nursing intervention, the impact of an intervention from the perspective of the patient, or the feasibility of the intervention in relation to cultural or organisational issues, systematic reviews and randomised controlled trials will always produce the best evidence on which to base practice, simply because they offer the best guarantee of validity and reliability.

For other nurses, however, different clinical issues are best served by different kinds of research evidence. For example, DiCenso *et al.* (1998 p. 39) argued that:

> *'Just as randomised trials and systematic overviews are the best designs for evaluating nursing interventions, qualitative studies are the best designs to better understand patients' experiences, attitudes and beliefs.*

DiCenso *et al.* acknowledge that their brand of EBP is based largely on David Sackett's writing about evidence-based *medicine* (Sackett *et al.*

1996), and that the RCT remains the gold standard for making decisions about which nursing intervention to employ, although we can see that they do accept that qualitative research findings might be more appropriate when the nurse needs to understand the experiences of individual patients.

We have already seen that other writers such as Anne Mulhall argue that nursing needs to distance itself from medicine, since 'in their operation, practice and culture, nursing and medicine remain quite different' (Mulhall 1998 p. 4). These writers often point out that whilst medicine is concerned primarily with cure, the role of the nurse is to care, and whilst cure is best measured using quantitative data, the measurement of care is far less clear-cut, if not impossible. Thus, Mulhall argues that nursing is concerned with 'untidy' things such as emotions and feelings, which are not amenable to quantitative scientific research and that qualitative research methodologies such as phenomenology and ethnography should stand alongside the RCT as equally valid and important.

Summary

- Some nurses regard evidence-based nursing as following the lead of evidence-based medicine by applying the findings from randomised controlled trials and other experimental research to *all* nursing problems.
- Others believe that *some* nursing issues are best resolved through the application of qualitative research findings.
- Others argue that just as nursing has a different agenda from medicine, so EBN should establish its own gold standards for judging research evidence.

Other forms of evidence

Clearly, research plays a major role in EBP and, for some, 'evidence-based practice is just another term for research usage' (Ingersoll 2000 p. 151). For most writers, however, evidence-based practice consists of far more than simply the application of the findings from research, whether quantitative or qualitative, and entails a number of other factors.

A good place to start investigating what else might go into an evidence-based decision might be with the much-quoted definition offered by David Sackett, a medical doctor and one of the founding members of the Evidence-Based Medicine Working Group. For Sackett: 'the practice of evidence-based medicine means integrating individual expertise with the best available external clinical evidence from systematic research' (Sackett *et al.* 1996 p. 71).

Whilst Sackett was quite clear that the RCT was the gold standard for external clinical evidence from research, he also maintained that research findings alone were not strong enough grounds on which to base a clinical decision. Somehow (and unfortunately, he does not make it clear exactly how), the practitioner must combine the research findings with 'individual expertise', which he described as 'the proficiency and judgement that individual clinicians acquire through clinical experience and clinical practice' (Sackett 1996 p. 71). For Sackett, then, EBP is more than simply another name for research-based practice; it is more than the mechanical process of applying the 'best evidence' regardless of the individual clinical situation; and entails a clinical judgement based upon a combination of gold standard research and clinical experience.

The frequency with which this definition is quoted in the nursing literature would suggest that many nurses are happy to accept that the practice of evidence-based nursing should broadly follow the lead of evidence-based medicine. However, DiCenso *et al.* later expanded this definition specifically for nursing, describing evidence-based nursing as: 'the process by which nurses make clinical decisions using the best available research evidence, their clinical expertise and patient preferences, in the context of available resources' (DiCenso *et al.* 1998 p. 38).

We have already seen that DiCenso *et al.* wished to expand the gold standard research methodology from RCTs in certain situations to include qualitative studies. We can also see that they regard EBP as comprising not only research and clinical expertise, but also 'patient preferences' and 'available resources' as two additional factors.

DiCenso *et al.* gave as an example of 'patient preferences', a patient who 'declines a treatment that clinical circumstances and research evidence indicate is best for his condition' (DiCenso *et al.* 1998 p. 38). We might argue, however, that this actually adds nothing to the definition, since patients always have the right to decline treatment. However, other writers take a far more positive meaning of the term 'patient preferences' as actively involving patients in decisions about their care, in keeping with the Government's notion of the 'expert patient'.

With regard to the issue of resources, DiCenso *et al.* cautioned that resource implications mean that the benefit of an intervention is sometimes outweighed by its costs. In other words, evidence-based decisions are constrained by financial and other restrictions, leading to possible compromises in what might otherwise be seen as best practice. Whilst DiCenso *et al.* seem to regard this as a basic fact of life, other writers warn that EBP might be used deliberately to restrict the number of interventions available to nurses, and could thus act as a justification for cost-cutting (White 1997 p. 178). In contrast, Sackett claimed that:

'Doctors practising evidence-based medicine will identify and apply the most efficacious interventions to maximise the quality and quantity of

life for individual patients; this may raise rather than lower the cost of their care.' (Sackett *et al* 1996 p. 72)

It would appear, then, that Sackett disagrees with the view that resource implications should be a factor in evidence-based decisions, preferring to regard EBP as an argument *against* cost-cutting.

Other writers have expanded the list of what might count as evidence. For example, some nurses take a more patient-centred approach in which 'best evidence' cannot be predetermined, but arises in response to the unique demands of each individual clinical situation (Mulhall 1998; French 1999; Hewitt-Taylor 2003). For these writers, the scope of what counts as evidence is often extended beyond the usual empirical sources, and might even include 'non-professional life experience' (Mulhall 1998 p. 5) or common sense. In a similar vein, le May (2000 p. 2) includes:

- evidence from research (either our own or others')
- evidence based on experiences (professional and general)
- evidence based on theory that is not research-based
- evidence gathered from clients/patients and/or their carers
- evidence passed on by role models/experts
- evidence based on policy directives.

However, expanding the scope of what might count as evidence brings with it a number of problems. First, these sources of evidence need to be appraised, since, as le May (2000 p. 6) points out, 'only the best available evidence will be used in practice'. What is not clear, however, is how such diverse sources of evidence are to be judged against one another. Second, the evidence must be implemented in practice. As le May (2000 p. 2) quite rightly points out:

> *'The complexity and skill of nursing, midwifery and health visiting relies on being able to fit together pieces of evidence collected from a variety of different sources in the quest for the total picture and resultant clinical effectiveness.'*

Unfortunately, it is very difficult to find any useful guidance as to how these various pieces might be judged and fitted together, beyond the vague notion that it involves some form of clinical judgement (Figure 5.1).

Whilst writers such as le May regard the expansion of what is to count as evidence in a positive light, others are more cautious. As Gerrish (2003 p. 107) pointed out:

> *'Simplistic definitions of evidence-based practice that state that research evidence is to be integrated with clinical expertise and patient preference fail to provide a clear indication of what is involved.'*

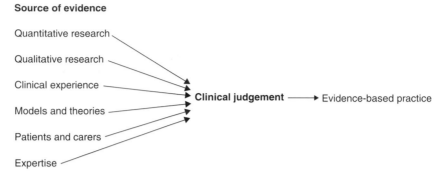

Figure 5.1 The role of clinical judgement in evidenced-based practice.

Peter French is also sceptical about the proliferation of different sources of evidence, and has identified five distinct uses of the term in the literature, which he summarises as:

- evidence as truth
- evidence as knowledge (including tacit knowledge, expert opinion and experiential knowledge)
- evidence as any relevant information that confirms or refutes a belief
- evidence as primary research findings
- evidence as meta-analyses and systematic reviews (French 2002 p. 254).

Rather than being complementary, French regarded these different views of evidence as conflicting with one another; rather than leading us towards a general and widely accepted single view of EBP, French argued that they signalled a fragmentation. Thus, he pointed out, 'in the final analysis it seems that EBP symbolism lacks consensus and that there is very little evidence to support the contention that a new construct or process exists' (French 2002 p. 255).

Summary

- Definitions of what counts as evidence have expanded over the years from the findings of research to a wide range of other factors.
- The difficulty with this expansion is that it becomes increasingly hard to make judgements about their relative value and how they might be combined.
- Whereas some writers regard this expansion of sources of evidence in a positive light, others argue that it indicates a lack of consensus about EBP.

Activity

How does the discussion about different types of evidence match with the ideas you had about evidence before you read this section?
How would you judge between different sources, and types, or evidence?

Hierarchies of evidence

We have seen that as we broaden out the ranges of evidence on which to base our practice, we are increasingly faced with the problem of how to evaluate their relative importance and how to make judgements between them. This is particularly problematic when different sources of evidence seem to indicate different courses of action. For example, many nurses will be able to recall situations where the research evidence pointed to one particular clinical decision and yet their experience or intuition suggested the opposite. In cases such as these, we need to know which source of evidence should take precedence: should we act according to the research or according to our own expertise?

One of the earliest responses to this problem was to elevate certain sources of evidence to gold standard status. In the very first published paper on evidence-based medicine, the Evidence-Based Medicine Working Group (EBMWG) clearly identified the RCT as the gold standard for practice, suggesting that only in situations where there is no evidence from RCTs 'one must fall back on weaker evidence' (EBMWG 1992 p. 2424). For many present-day writers from both medicine and nursing, the RCT and, more recently, the systematic review of several RCTs, continues to have gold standard status.

More recently, however, the idea of a gold standard has been expanded into a complete hierarchy which ranks all sources of evidence according to their merit. A number of such hierarchies have been published over the past few years, of which four specific to nursing and midwifery are reproduced in Table 5.2.

Although at first sight, all four hierarchies might seem very similar, a closer inspection will reveal some interesting differences. The top of all four hierarchies are, in fact, almost identical, with each having RCTs and other experimental research or else systematic reviews of several RCTs as the gold standard. Despite a number of reassuring remarks that evidence-based nursing places a high value on qualitative research findings, all of the hierarchies would appear to suggest otherwise. Indeed, an examination of Evans' hierarchy appears to suggest that descriptive studies and case studies are, by definition, studies of poor methodological quality.

However, it is at the bottom end of the hierarchies that some interesting differences appear. Two of the four hierarchies rate expert

Table 5.2 Hierarchies of evidence.

Ellis (2000)	Aslam (2000)	Evans (2003)	Norman and Ryrie (2004)
(1) systematic reviews (2) large-scale well-designed primary studies, RCTs and other controlled trials (3) large-scale primary studies using other methodologies (4a) descriptive studies and reports (4b) opinions and experience of respected authorities based on clinical experience and professional consensus	(1) randomised controlled testing (2) controlled testing on selected groups (3) non-controlled testing (4) testing on selected small samples (5) tests carried out outside a formal research environment (6) personal experience (7) clinical tradition (8) anecdotes	(1) systematic reviews, multi-centre studies (2) RCT, observational studies (3) uncontrolled trials with dramatic results, before and after studies, non-randomised controlled trials (4) descriptive studies, case studies, expert opinion, studies of poor methodological quality	(1) systematic reviews (2) RCTs (3) well-designed intervention studies without randomisation (4) well-designed observation studies (5) expert opinion, including the opinion of service users and carers

opinion as the lowest form of evidence. Of these, one includes the opinion of service users and carers as having equal status to that of nurses (Norman and Ryrie 2004), whilst the other gives equal status to expert opinion, descriptive studies, case studies and 'studies of poor methodological quality' (Evans 2003). A third hierarchy gives bottom place to 'opinions and experiences of respected authorities based on clinical experience and professional consensus' (Ellis 2000), whilst the fourth places both clinical tradition and anecdotes below personal experience (Aslam 2000).

We might, therefore, begin to ask ourselves how the use of hierarchies can be reconciled with the earlier views of Sackett, DiCenso, le May and others that an evidence-based decision entails a combination of many different types of evidence. Are these writers suggesting that evidence from qualitative studies, clinical expertise, patient preferences, resource implications, personal experience and so on be given equal status to evidence from RCTs, that evidence from these other sources should be given either higher or lower status, or that it should only be employed when no RCTs have been conducted?

Summary

- Hierarchies of evidence have been created in an effort to help nurses distinguish between sources.
- These might, however, serve to confuse, rather than clarify the issue of what is good evidence.

Judging evidence for use in practice

Judgements based on hierarchies

The rather confusing answer to the above question is that all of these suggestions have been made by different writers at some point over the past fifteen years. As we have seen, the first published paper on evidence-based medicine asserted that, wherever possible, practice should be based on findings from RCTs, and only in cases where there was no gold standard research evidence should the practitioner look to other sources such as 'intuition, unsystematic clinical experience and pathophysiologic rationale' (EBMWG 1992 p. 2420). In a later paper, Sackett *et al.* (1996 p. 72) echoed this position when they awarded gold standard status to the RCT and instructed that: 'if no randomised trial has been carried out for our patient's predicament, we must follow the trail to the next best external evidence and work from there.' Only in cases where there is no research evidence at all should decisions be based on non-research-based evidence such as 'opinions of respected authorities'.

Rolfe and Gardner (2006) refer to this approach to EBP as the 'exclusive hierarchy' model, in which practitioners start at the top and work their way down until they find the 'best evidence' on which to base their practice. And whilst the 'exclusive hierarchy' approach might be simplest to implement, other writers, particularly in the field of nursing, have suggested that practitioners should employ an 'inclusive hierarchy' model in which all sources of evidence are considered together, but those higher in the hierarchy are given more weighting than those lower down (Aslam 2000; Hewitt-Taylor 2003). Other writers argue that different hierarchies should be produced for *different types* of clinical problems (Evans 2003), or that *each individual problem* should be judged on its own merits (Mulhall 1998).

Yet others appear to be completely confused about the issue of hierarchies of evidence, and have expressed conflicting views in the same paper. For example, Ellis (2000), in describing her benchmarking project, stated variously that 'the evidence base . . . was considered continuously using a hierarchy of evidence' (p. 215); that she had 'not used a hierarchy to categorise evidence but [had] approached the classification of evidence without overt value judgements' (p. 219); that 'using lower level evidence is only accepted in the absence of more empirical, higher level evidence' (p. 218); and that 'evidence is . . . considered from any level of the hierarchy' (p. 218). The situation is probably best summed up by Rycroft-Malone *et al.* (2004 p. 87–88), who concluded that:

> *'Agreed standards for determining whether research evidence is appropriate and useful for a particular patient/context and how it can be used have yet to be developed . . . How these sources are melded together in the real-time of clinical decision-making is still virtually unknown.'*

Thus, despite a great deal of general advice about combining or integrating evidence from different levels of the hierarchy, very little has been written about how the nurse should go about this complex task.

Summary

- Almost all hierarchies of evidence place findings from quantitative research at the top, and qualitative research and expert opinion at the bottom.
- In general, there is a great deal of confusion surrounding the use of these hierarchies.
- Some writers argue for an 'exclusive' model in which only the 'best' evidence is used.
- Others prefer an 'inclusive' model in which all evidence is weighted according to its position.
- Yet others argue that different hierarchies should be produced for different nursing issues, or that each issue should be judged on its own merits.

If EBP was merely a case of somehow making judgements about evidence based on its position in a hierarchy the issue would be complex enough, but unfortunately there is also the issue of expertise to consider.

Judgements based on expertise

If we look again at the hierarchies in Table 5.2, we will see that three of them explicitly include expert opinion at the very bottom, and the other two refer to clinical and personal experience, also as a very lowly form of evidence. Such a low placing on the hierarchy is consistent with the previously discussed view of EBP that 'de-emphasises intuition, unsystematic clinical experience and pathophysiologic rationale' (EBMWG 1992) in favour of research-based evidence. However, we have also seen that not all writers agree with this view. White, for example, appears to want to turn the hierarchy on its head when she writes:

'Perhaps **the most obviously flawed assumption** is that examining research using RCTs is the best way to evaluate the effectiveness of interventions and a better basis for clinical decision-making than the clinical experience of the practitioner.' (White 1997 p. 177, my emphasis)

McKenna *et al.* (2000) go even further, claiming that basing clinical decisions according to the findings from research is both naïve and foolish:

'Many nurses erroneously believe that all practice should be based on research. The desire to achieve this has been shown to be naïve and foolish. The view that when good evidence exists one should automatically use it, is equally naïve: nurses might legitimately use ethical evidence, aesthetic evidence or personal evidence to justify ignoring the use of existing empirical evidence, as long as they remain professionally and personally accountable for their actions.' (McKenna et al. 2000 p. 42)

This view is in stark contrast to that of Ellis (2000 pp. 217–218), who argued that such 'individual responsibility' and 'total freedom of decision-making' is potentially dangerous for both patients and practitioners, and claimed instead that where clear and unequivocal evidence exists, 'there is no room for discussion or compromise'.

However, the situation is not as black and white as it might first appear. It is not simply a dispute between those (often medical) writers who argue that expertise should be at the bottom of the hierarchy and those (mainly nursing) writers who believe it should be at the top. The problem is that, on the one hand, writers such as Sackett and DiCenso suggest that EBP entails a *combination* of evidence from gold standard research alongside the individual expertise of the practitioner, whilst on the other hand, most of the hierarchies of evidence appear to rate clinical experience and expertise 'as the lowest level of evidence' (Evans 2003 p. 81). It is perhaps difficult to see how these writers can be advocating at the same time that we should always use 'best evidence' *and* that we should use evidence from the bottom of the hierarchy. The situation is made even more confusing by Sackett's further assertion that:

'External clinical evidence [from research] can inform, but can never replace, individual clinical expertise, **and it is this expertise that decides whether the external evidence applies to the individual patient at all** and, if so, how it should be integrated into a clinical decision.' (Sackett et al. 1996 p. 72, my emphasis)

What Sackett appears to be saying is that evidence from the bottom of the hierarchy can always override evidence from the top, which calls into question the very purpose of having a hierarchy in the first place, and suggests that expertise is a more effective basis for practice than the findings from empirical research.

Such a view appears directly to contradict the basic ethos of EBP, that clinical decisions should be based upon the best evidence from research rather than on the unreliable and subjective experience of the practitioner. Indeed, we have already seen that the original rationale for evidence-based medicine was to devalue the experience of experts (Davidoff *et al.* 1995) and to 'put a much lower value on [clinical] authority' (EBMWG 1992 p. 2421).

Some nurses are very concerned by the approach to EBP that seeks to devalue clinical authority and expertise, and point out that any move to de-emphasise intuition and clinical experience also devalues the expert practitioner in favour of the blind application of the findings from experimental research. These practitioners find such a thought quite disturbing, since it suggests that the most important determinant of good practice is not how much experience and/or expertise nurses possess, but how many research journals they have read.

Perhaps the most famous advocate of clinical expertise is the American nurse academic Patricia Benner. Benner's work, particularly her seminal book *From Novice to Expert* (Benner 1984), argues strongly that the use of so-called gold standard evidence from the top of the hierarchy is a characteristic of novice practice. In contrast, Benner argues that expert nurses rarely base their practice on the published findings of research, relying instead on their 'intuitive grasp' of the situation. Dreyfus and Dreyfus, on whose work Benner drew heavily, made the same point with regard to medicine:

> '*In reality, a patient is viewed by the experienced doctor as a unique case and treated on the basis of intuitively perceived similarity with situations previously encountered. That kind of wisdom, unfortunately, cannot be shared and thereby made the basis of a doctor's rational decision.*'
> (Dreyfus and Dreyfus 1986)

Such a view of expertise has a number of important implications for evidence-based practice. First, clinical expertise, which Sackett argued should be the mechanism for deciding whether and how research findings should be applied to practice, is not a rational process; and second, it cannot be put into words. If there is an evidence-base for expert practice, it is personal and tacit.

We are now a very long way from Ingersoll's view, cited earlier, that EBP is just another term for research usage. However, although we have seen that there are many other kinds of evidence apart from research findings, we are no further on in our understanding of how these different types of evidence are brought together in an evidence-based judgement, or indeed, whether such judgements can ever be the subject of rational scrutiny.

Summary

- Most writers agree that expertise has an important role to play in EBP.
- Some, including Sackett, claim that expertise is the deciding factor in evidence-based decisions.
- However, Benner claims that expert decisions are not open to rational scrutiny.

Activity

Where do you stand in this debate?
How would you weigh up the use of clinical expertise against rational evidence from research findings?

Using evidence to support decisions in practice

Let us now return to Sackett's definition of EBP as integrating individual expertise with the best available research evidence. First, we have seen that there is a great deal of dispute about how we make judgements about which research evidence is best for any given clinical situation; whether what is 'best' for medicine is necessarily 'best' for nursing; whether the same type of evidence is best for all clinical situations; and whether we should accept forms of evidence other than that arising from research. Second, we have seen that some writers regard 'individual expertise' as a poor form of evidence, which then makes it difficult to accept Sackett's injunction that it is this expertise which decides 'whether the external [research] evidence applies to the individual patient at all' (Sackett *et al.* 1996 p. 72).

In fact, Sackett's view that clinical expertise can always override the evidence from research only makes sense if expertise is taken out of the hierarchy of evidence. In this scenario, expertise would no longer be regarded as a lowly form of evidence, equivalent to anecdotes and poorly designed studies, but would instead form the very basis of the clinical judgement about whether and/or how to apply the evidence (see Figure 5.2).

This view of the role of expertise has some important implications for evidence-based practice, particularly if we accept Benner's position that expertise is not the result of a conscious decision-making process and often cannot even be articulated, since it suggests that evidence-based practice is not the rational, scientific process that it is sometimes made out to be.

It is perhaps this role of expertise in EBP that highlights the crucial differences between evidence-based *medicine* and evidence-based

Source of evidence

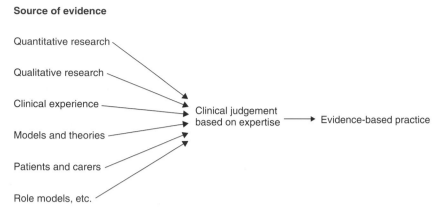

Figure 5.2 Expertise as a form of clinical judgement.

nursing. The issue is brought into sharp relief by the definition of evidence-based medicine offered by Greenhalgh (2006 p. 1) as: 'the use of figures [statistics] derived from research on *populations* to inform decisions about *individuals.*' As Rolfe (1999) has pointed out, this argument only holds true if all individuals in the population respond in much the same way. So, for example, evidence about the effectiveness of a new drug can be deduced from a population study to individual patients because it is assumed that most individuals will respond in more or less the same way to the same medication. However, many nurses believe that 'nursing consists of interactions between unique individuals, with unique experiences, and it always takes place in unique situations' (Sarvimaki 1988). If that is indeed the case, then the outcomes of nursing interventions are not predictable in the same way as medical interventions, and we can never be sure that the *general* findings from RCTs and other statistically-based research methodologies will tell us anything about any *particular* nursing encounter.

Perhaps we should simply accept that there can be no formula for making clinical nursing judgements, no rational process for arriving at the right answer or 'best practice' that works on every occasion. Or perhaps we might argue for two distinct and different forms of evidence-based practice.

On the one hand, some nursing interventions, particularly at the more medical end of the spectrum, would benefit from *the science of finding, evaluating, and implementing the results of medical research'* (Greenhalgh 2006 p. xiii) which employs:

'The use of mathematical estimates of the risk of benefit and harm, derived from high quality research on population samples, to inform clinical decision-making in the diagnosis, investigation or management of individual patients.' (Greenhalgh 2006 p. 1)

When nurses make evidence-based decisions in these clinical situations, they would do well to pay attention to the findings of RCTs, and to make decisions based on exclusive hierarchies of evidence which evaluate research findings in terms of the validity and reliability of the methods used to generate them.

On the other hand, however, many nursing interventions would also benefit from regarding nursing as a *'science of the unique'* (Rolfe and Gardner 2005 p. 297) which is: 'based on the premise that nursing is a series of individual and unique encounters which cannot be described by a science of large numbers.'

In these cases, findings from generalisable research cannot be counted upon to provide nurses with reliable information on which to make judgements about the unique clinical situations they find themselves in. What is required here is a more intimate, personal and intuitive form of decision-making based on the expertise of the nurse and their personal knowledge about the individual patient.

Chapter summary

The first paper outlining the principles of evidence-based medicine was published in 1992, and after only three, Davidoff *et al.* (1995) were asking 'why all the fuss?' and arguing that EBM was so obviously the route to best practice that they could not see how anyone could object to it. However, early attempts to apply the principles of EBM to nursing met with some strong objections by those who saw the role of the nurse as very different to that of the doctor, and we have spent the past decade attempting to clarify exactly how nurses might work within an evidence-based framework. Whilst some nurses have concluded that the most promising route is to follow the lead of our medical colleagues, others have argued for a far broader approach which encompasses not only evidence from qualitative research, but also reflective practice and expertise. The ensuing claims and counter-claims have led at least one writer to question whether we can claim that evidence-based practice even exists as a viable concept. Thus, ten years after the Evidence-Based Medicine Working Group proclaimed that 'a new paradigm for medical practice is emerging' (EBMWG 1992 p. 2420), Peter French was moved to conclude that: 'in the final analysis it seems that EBP symbolism lacks consensus and that there is very little evidence to support the contention that a new construct or process exists' (French 2002 p. 255).

In this chapter I have outlined and explored some of the many ways that nursing and medical writers have tried to describe and explain EBP since that initial publication in 1992. I have not attempted, as some other writers have tried, to arrive at a definition or general account of evidence-based practice, but rather I have concluded that different approaches might suit different nursing situations, from the rigid 'exclusive hierarchy' approach at one extreme to the intuitive expertise approach at the other.

The aim of this chapter has therefore not been to tell you what EBP is, or (even more difficult) to tell you how to do it. Rather, I hope that it has helped you to think for yourself what it might mean for you and your practice, and to inspire you to read about and discuss this most difficult and important of issues in wider and deeper detail.

References

Aslam, R. (2000) Research and evidence in midwifery. In: Proctor, S. and Renfrew, M. (ed.) *Linking Research and Practice in Midwifery: A Guide to Evidence-Based Practice* (pp. 15–34). Baillière Tindall, Edinburgh.

Benner, P. (1984) *From Novice to Expert: Excellence and Power in Clinical Nursing Practice*. Addison-Wesley, Menlo Park.

Davidoff, F., Case, K. and Fried, P.W. (1995) Evidence-based medicine: why all the fuss? *Annals of Internal Medicine*, **122** (9), 727.

DiCenso, A., Cullum, N. and Ciliska, D. (1998) Implementing evidence-based nursing: some misconceptions. *Evidence-based Nursing*, **1** (2), 38–40.

Dreyfus, H.L. and Dreyfus, S.E. (1986) *Mind Over Machine*. Blackwell Publishing, Oxford.

Ellis, J. (2000) Sharing the evidence: clinical practice benchmarking to improve continuously the quality of care. *Journal of Advanced Nursing*, **32** (1), 215–225.

Evans, D. (2003) Hierarchy of evidence: a framework for ranking evidence evaluating health care interventions. *Journal of Clinical Nursing*, **12**, 77–84.

Evidence-Based Medicine Working Group (1992) Evidence-based medicine: a new approach to teaching the practice of medicine. *Journal of American Medical Association*, **268** (17), 2420–2425.

Feinstein, A. and Horwitz, R. (1997) Problems in the 'evidence' of 'evidence-based medicine'. *American Journal of Medicine*, **103**, 529–535.

French, P. (1999) The development of evidence-based nursing. *Journal of Advanced Nursing*, **29** (1), 72–78.

French, P. (2002) What is the evidence on evidence-based practice? An epistemological concern. *Journal of Advanced Nursing*, **37** (3), 250–257.

Gerrish, K. (2003) Evidence-based practice: unravelling the rhetoric and making it real. *Practice Development in Health Care*, **2** (2), 99–113.

Greenhalgh, T. (2006) *How to Read a Paper: The Basics of Evidence-based Medicine* (3rd edn). BMJ Publishing Group, London.

Hewitt-Taylor, J. (2003) Reviewing evidence. *Intensive and Critical Care Nursing*, **19**, 43–49.

Ingersoll, G.L. (2000) Evidence-based nursing: what it is and what it isn't. *Nursing Outlook*, **48**, 151–152.

le May, A. (2000) Evidence-based practice. *Nursing Times Clinical Monographs*, **1**.

McKenna, H., Cutcliffe, J. and McKenna, P. (2000) Evidence-based practice – demolishing some myths. *Nursing Standard*, **14** (16), 39–42.

Mulhall, A. (1998) Nursing, research and the evidence. *Evidence-based Nursing*, **1** (1), 4–6.

Norman, I. and Ryrie, I. (2004) *The Art and Science of Mental Health Nursing.* Open University Press, Maidenhead.

Rolfe, G. (1999) Insufficient evidence: the problems of evidence-based medicine. *Nurse Education Today*, **19**, 422–442.

Rolfe, G. and Gardner, L. (2005) Towards a nursing science of the unique: evidence, reflexivity and the study of persons. *Journal of Research in Nursing*, **10** (3), 297–310.

Rolfe, G. and Gardner, L. (2006) Towards a geology of evidence-based practice – a discussion paper. *International Journal of Nursing Studies* (in press).

Rycroft-Malone, J., Seers, K., Titchen, A., Harvey, G., Kitson, A. and McCormack, B. (2004) What counts as evidence in evidence-based practice? *Journal of Advanced Nursing*, **47** (1), 81–90.

Sackett, D., Rosenberg, W., Gray, J., Haynes, R. and Richardson, W. (1996) Evidence-based medicine: what it is and what it isn't. *British Journal of Medicine*, **312**, 71–72.

Sarvimaki, A. (1988) Nursing as a moral, practical, communicative and creative activity. *Journal of Advanced Nursing*, **13**, 462–467.

White, A.J. (1997) Evidence-based practice and nursing: the new panacea? *British Journal of Nursing*, **6** (3), 175–178.

6
Portfolios and the use of evidence

Learning objectives

This chapter explores how portfolios can be used to support and demonstrate learning and development from both a pre-registration and a post-qualifying point of view. Portfolios are always constructed with a specific purpose in mind; successful portfolios are structured to meet this purpose, and their contents are selected to demonstrate the achievement of learning objectives, outcomes or the demonstration of competence and fitness for practice. This chapter considers different frameworks for portfolio construction and introduces the reader to strategies for portfolio development. Key to portfolio construction is the creation of evidence and the use of reflective writing to demonstrate the qualities of the practitioner.

By the end of this chapter you will have:

- an understanding of the nature of a portfolio
- explored a range of structures to be used in compiling a portfolio
- an understanding of the requirements of a learning portfolio or one that meets Nursing and Midwifery Council requirements
- an understanding of how a portfolio can demonstrate competence as an accountable practitioner
- explored the nature of evidence used within portfolios
- considered creating portfolios using different techniques
- considered the ethical issues of constructing a portfolio.

What is a portfolio?

Defining a portfolio

A portfolio, when used in a professional context, is simply a collection of documents that present a picture of the practitioner. It is like a photo album, but in word, not visual, pictures. The commonest and most widely accepted definition of a portfolio is that by Brown (1995 p. 3) who identifies it as:

> *'A private collection of evidence which demonstrates the continuing acquisition of skills, knowledge, attitudes, understanding and achievements. It is both retrospective and prospective, as well as reflecting the current stage of development and activity of the individual.'*

This emphasises several features of portfolios:

- Their *individual* nature: portfolios are unique to the person compiling them and provide a permanent record of that person's professional history.
- They are *dynamic* in nature in that they reflect the past but anticipate and plan for the future.
- They document and record specific *attributes* of the individual concerned.
- They comprise various types of *evidence*.

However, McMullan *et al.* (2003 p. 288) added to this definition by suggesting that a portfolio is:

> *'A collection of evidence, usually in written form, of both the products and processes of learning. It attests to achievement and personal and professional development, by providing critical analysis of its contents.'*

This builds on Brown's (1995) definition by acknowledging the value of exploring *how* attributes have been gained, as opposed to simply establishing that they have. Similarly, McMullan *et al.* (2003) identify the cognitive processes involved in using a portfolio as a learning tool by referring to the analysis that takes place within a dynamic and living process of construction. This moves the concept of a portfolio on from being a recording device, to one of activity and interaction used on a continuous basis through a practitioner's life.

Qualified nurses' use of portfolios

The demonstration of professional competence is a crucial element of being a registered, accountable practitioner. The Nursing and Midwifery Council requires all practitioners on its live register to compile an ongoing portfolio to demonstrate their fitness to remain eligible to practise. Although this is seen as the responsibility of the individual practitioner and it is taken on trust that all will do so, a 5% sample of people re-registering every three years will have their portfolios audited to ensure they comply with the minimum requirements for Post-Registration Education and Practice (PREP) (NMC 2004a).

The components of the portfolio are not specified by the NMC, but an assumption is made that the practitioner will construct a portfolio that demonstrates fitness to practise, and contains evidence that shows how the requirements for ongoing registration have been met.

Clearly then, the construction of a professional portfolio brings together all of the elements covered in this book so far. To a large extent a successful and convincing portfolio is dependent on the practitioner having developed reflective skills and competence in reflective writing so that they can show how new knowledge is created from and incorporated into their practice.

Students' use of portfolios

Students on the majority of pre-registration courses will be introduced to portfolio construction within their programme of study. Other practitioners engaging in continuing professional development activity are also likely to have to produce a portfolio at some stage in their course. These portfolios are specifically designed to demonstrate the acquisition and development of competence and are essentially learning portfolios whose purpose is to demonstrate the achievement of specified learning outcomes. These portfolios are usually subjected to objective assessment by others who are in a position to make a judgement about the contents according to pre-specified criteria. Pre-registration and/or course portfolios are therefore different in their focus to those compiled by registered practitioners where the primary purpose is in demonstrating fitness for continuing practice. The registered practitioner therefore needs to provide evidence of their own continuing development and their commitment to evidence-based practice.

Summary

- Professional portfolios are collections of documents that paint a picture of the practitioner for a particular purpose.
- They are individual in nature.
- They present a record of the practitioner's professional history and achievements.
- They are dynamic in nature and constructed throughout a practitioner's working life.
- They record the attributes of the practitioner.
- They comprise various types of evidence.

- Student portfolios are usually constructed for the purposes of learning and demonstrating achievement of competencies and learning outcomes.
- Qualified practitioners' portfolios are constructed to demonstrate their fitness to practise in fulfilment of the requirements of the NMC for triennial registration.
- Portfolios may include the practitioner's personal development plan.

Activity

Identify the reason you are putting together a portfolio. What is it you want it to demonstrate?

The purpose of a portfolio

A portfolio is always kept for a particular purpose, and everything concerned with the portfolio, from the structure you use to organise it, its content, and the ethical issues related to it, derive from this purpose. Some of these purposes are shown in Table 6.1.

It is easy to begin collecting material for your portfolio without being clear what, exactly, the purpose of your portfolio is. However, this is not the most effective or efficient way of going about things as it could mean that you include lots of material that is not related to the reason why you are compiling the portfolio. This may result in you spending

Table 6.1   Purposes of portfolio construction.

As a student	As a registered practitioner
For assessment purposes	To demonstrate your competence and fitness to practise
As an ongoing record of your progress and achievements	To fulfil NMC requirements for PREP
To demonstrate your development as a practitioner	To provide evidence of your accountability as a practitioner
As a self-directed log of your activities	As an ongoing record of your development as a practitioner
As a guide for your self-directed learning	As a way of working through and documenting your experiences
As a tool to document reflective learning and practice	As a requirement for annual appraisal with your employer
As part of your personal development plan	In preparation for a new job application
	As part of your personal development plan

a lot of extra time on it without focusing on what you are trying to achieve. Compare this to the way you would prepare for carrying out a work-based task, such as doing a dressing. Before taking your equipment to the patient's bedside, you would first have worked out what you would need and gone through, in your head, the process to be used to ensure that you selected the appropriate equipment needed to complete the task. What you would not do is to overload your trolley with every dressing pack and piece of equipment available in the clinical room.

It is also important to remember that what goes into your portfolio is under your control; you choose the content. No one else can require you to put in your portfolio what you do not consider to be in your best interest. To use the analogy of the photograph album again, you would not put an unflattering picture of yourself in your album; you'd either find better ones, or leave out the images completely. So, in terms of what goes into your portfolio, it is up to you to present the picture or yourself as the practitioner you think you are. You do not have to illustrate your weaknesses, unless you want to show how you have addressed these and developed in a professional way as a result. Whilst identifying areas for improvement are a very positive way of tackling our professional development, it is only worth including these in a portfolio if they also demonstrate a positive outcome.

So, it is important to establish the boundaries and parameters you need to work within to achieve what is needed from the very beginning of your portfolio work. For instance, you need to consider:

- What particular *picture* of you as a practitioner do you want the portfolio to paint?
- Who will see the portfolio?
- What part of it is a *public* document, as opposed to the part that is kept private and for your own use?
- What does it need to contain; that is, what are the essential or specified components that have to be present for this specific purpose?
- What are the criteria that it will be judged against, for example marking criteria, PREP criteria, PDP, learning objectives or outcomes?
- What length does it need to be? Which parts of it contribute to the word count? Very often it is only the original written material that counts within the wordage, not the evidence used to support these.
- When do you need to have it written by? Do you have a specific timeframe to work to which limits the scope of what you can present or within which you need to complete the components, such as practice assessment tools?

The 5WH cues are useful here in helping you to frame the questions about the purpose of your portfolio.

Activity

Establish the boundaries and parameters that apply to your own portfolio by working through the questions in the section above.

Summary

- Portfolios are always constructed for a particular purpose.
- Planning your portfolio to achieve this purpose is essential.

Structuring a portfolio

The portfolio may simply be a collection of papers that are conveniently kept together in one place. On the other hand, a portfolio may have a complex structure and be organised through a series of sections; each section may contain a selection of material depending on what it is designed to demonstrate. Hence, there are many ways a portfolio can be constructed provided it fulfils the purpose it is being compiled for.

Qualified practitioners have a carte blanche to use whatever structure for a portfolio they find most useful and to suit their own professional needs. Some employers issue a portfolio format to all their employees. These often contain a personal development plan in addition to sections for filing such things as certificates, course attendance, training days and other evidence of professional development.

Students are often provided with templates for portfolios to ensure the learning outcomes and competencies they are expected to achieve are the guiding components for its compilation. These may derive from the philosophy of the curriculum or assessment strategy running throughout the programme and reflect both the theoretical content and practical competencies. These enable students to develop the experience and skills of compiling a portfolio without the added stress of needing to devise a structure for them.

However, in post-qualifying courses, open or work-based learning modules, portfolios may be used to enable students to study diverse topics and build their knowledge and skills base within their own specialties of practice. Portfolios for this type of module are usually devised by the student themselves, using a guiding learning contract that is negotiated and agreed with an academic supervisor. This has the advantage of enabling practitioners to specify their own learning needs, devise an action and study plan to achieve these, and construct the portfolio to demonstrate them. Clearly, a pre-written template will not be appropriate in these circumstances.

The very basic components of a portfolio are the objectives or outcomes that the portfolio is being constructed to demonstrate and the evidence that is used to support their achievement.

Summary

- The guiding principle for devising a portfolio structure is that it fulfils the purpose it is constructed for.
- Students are usually provided with a portfolio structure to ensure learning outcomes and competencies are achieved.
- Open and work-based modules may require the student to devise their own portfolio structure under the supervision of their academic tutor.
- Qualified practitioners have scope to construct their own portfolios or use prefabricated ones.
- The basic components are the objectives or outcomes and the evidence used to demonstrate these.
- These components may be supplemented by reflective reviews and commentaries which link the evidence to the outcomes. These are more likely to be included in portfolios written at higher academic levels.

Defining the outcomes and setting objectives

If the purpose of the portfolio construction is clear, then it follows that the parameters and outcomes expected to be demonstrated within it will also be clearly specified. An outcome is a defined end point of what is to be achieved as a result of the activity undertaken, of which the portfolio construction is part. Objectives are specific goals to be achieved. Both outcomes and objectives need to be phrased in clear, unambivalent language to provide a baseline measure that the portfolio is tested against. For instance, if a learning outcome is phrased as 'to demonstrate competent skills in clinical nursing practice', the evidence presented to show this has been achieved has to illustrate that acquisition. Thus, the evidence may be on a clinical skills assessment tool, or a report from an assessor who has observed the student in practice. Hence, the clear identification of the outcomes or objectives should provide a logical path to determining what sort of evidence will be needed to confirm it has been achieved.

Summary

- Outcome statements define the parameters of the portfolio.
- Clearly defined outcome statements provide guidance for the type of evidence that will confirm their achievement.

Using evidence in a portfolio

The other crucial component of the portfolio is the evidence provided by the practitioner to demonstrate the claims they are making. Evidence can take many forms, but essentially it can be anything that 'proves' the point that you are trying to make. So, any evidence that is included in your portfolio needs to be linked to something else to show just what it is you are demonstrating. Table 6.2 gives some examples of the range of evidence that could be used to demonstrate a particular point.

It is important to remember that evidence cannot stand by itself; it has to be linked to the point it is supporting. This, in a way, is just like the use of evidence in a trial; a lawyer will not let the evidence stand by itself to tell a story. What he or she does instead is weave the evidence together in a particular way, drawing conclusions from it to make his or her case. Of course, another lawyer can challenge this interpretation, so it is the veracity of the evidence that is important, in terms of being credible, but it is the case that is being made using it that tells us what we need to know. It could be that one piece of evidence is used to illustrate or justify more than one particular achievement or aspect, so the creative use of evidence will cut down on the amount of paper needed in a portfolio.

So, in using evidence in a portfolio, it is not enough to simply include something such as a set of lecture notes and handouts, or to photocopy articles from a journal and hope that your reader knows what they are

Table 6.2 Examples of the range of evidence that may be used in a portfolio.

Outcome	Evidence that may be used to support achievement
Achieving a clinical competence	Records of carrying out the competence plus a signed statement from your assessor
Demonstrating evidence-based practice	A summary of the sources of evidence you have used and the conclusions reached An analysis of the element of practice with an assessment of what needs to change
Demonstrating patient-centred care	A copy of a care plan that you have devised for a patient
Demonstrating patient education	A copy of a patient information leaflet you have devised
Professional development	Attendance certificates at learning events and a written reflective review of what you have learnt and how this informs your practice

included for. What needs to happen is that every piece of evidence is mapped to an outcome, competence or achievement. It may also be further developed through a reflective review or commentary or cross-referencing. Any of the reflective writing techniques introduced in Chapter 3 can be used to do this.

Types of evidence

Evidence within a portfolio falls into two main types – *primary* and *secondary*.

Primary evidence is anything that is constructed by the practitioner for the purpose of the portfolio itself. For instance:

- reflective reviews
- consideration of achievement of learning outcomes
- commentaries on experiences
- written critical incident analysis
- notes of clinical supervision meetings.

Secondary evidence is, on the whole, already in existence, but is brought into the portfolio to support the claims that are being made. For instance:

- a curriculum vitae
- copies of patient information leaflets
- protocols developed
- letters or testimonials from others
- copies of articles written, or other publications
- reviews of work
- marking feedback sheets.

When deciding on what evidence to use in a portfolio, it is worth using the checklist in Box 6.1 to ensure it is both relevant and appropriate for the task you need it to perform.

Summary

- Evidence can be primary or secondary.
- Evidence does not stand alone to demonstrate anything. It needs to be linked to other components of the portfolio to demonstrate achievements.
- Evidence needs to be organised and referenced in some way.

Activity

Consider the evidence that you are using in your portfolio and test it against the checklist in Box 6.1.

Box 6.1 Checklist for selecting evidence to be used in a portfolio.

For each piece of evidence you are considering using ask yourself:

Is this primary or secondary evidence?
What is its purpose?
What does it demonstrate?
Which learning outcome/objective/assessment criteria or achievement does it relate to?
Can it be used to support or illustrate more than one point/achievement?
Which analytical point in the commentary/reflective review does it support?
How can I reference it in the text?
Where will I put it in the portfolio?

Models of portfolios

Over the past 15 years, since portfolios started to be used in nursing and midwifery education, there has been considerable development in the nature and diversity of portfolios found, both within education and professional practice itself. Endacott *et al.* (2004)[1] identified four approaches to portfolio construction, which increase in sophistication in both the content and processes involved in their compilation.

- **The shopping trolley model**: this is a collection of papers amassed during the time covered by the portfolio, such as handouts and lecture notes, photocopies of articles, practice assessment documents, and kept within a large folder. It has little analytical content or cohesion and little or no attempt at linking the evidence presented to the learning outcomes. In educational terms a portfolio like this is often a required component of the course but is not assessed in any way.
- **The toastrack model**: the portfolio consists of separate elements that assess different aspects of practice or theory, such as a skills log or a reflective account. The folder or binder in which they are kept acts as a convenient organiser using the required headings for assessment, but there is no overarching attempt at cohesion between the parts. Parts of the portfolio might be used for assessment.
- **The spinal column model**: this model is structured around practice competencies, with the competency forming the 'vertebra' and the supporting evidence slotted in to demonstrate how each

---

[1] This work was the result of a national study funded by the English National Board for Nurses, Midwives and Health Visitors exploring 'The use of portfolios in the assessment of learning and competence'.

competence is met. Analytical accounts are often included to show how theory informs practice, or reflective accounts of incidents or case studies support the achievement of the competencies as evidence. Narratives may link more than one competence together, demonstrating transference of knowledge and skills and the interpretation of elements of practice. The emphasis in this model is on the original work of the student in the narratives, with the evidence being used to support the case being made. This model of portfolio is always constructed for assessment purposes, with credit being awarded for the original work and supporting evidence supplied as verification.

- **The cake mix model**: in this model, the sum total of the parts it contains is seen to be more than the individual components in terms of what it demonstrates about the practitioner concerned. The emphasis is on the integration of all the parts within an overarching narrative which forms the basis of assessment. Only evidence that is referred to in the narrative is included, and the narrative tends to consist of a reflective account that incorporates elements of practice, theory, learning and the evidence itself. Thus, essential elements of the model are reflectivity, practice and professional development.

The use of these types of models within educational programmes loosely fits with the increase in academic level as the student progresses through their course. Certainly, the use of the cake mix model was found predominantly in programmes leading to advanced practice or Master's level. The toastrack model was more likely to be found where beginning students were being introduced to the notion of portfolios as collecting evidence to support the development of practice and the student's own expression of competence.

These models provide us with a useful guide for assessing our own portfolio and its structure against the objective criteria that will be used to measure or assess it. This gives us a guide to the structure of the portfolio which will best suit our purposes, and ensures that the contents match what we are trying to achieve. The case studies below show how decisions about portfolio structure can be made in this way, and using the models identified.

Case study 6.1 Creating a portfolio of evidence to demonstrate developing competence at level one using the 'toastrack' model.

Mark is a student nurse who is about to embark on his first clinical placement on a hospital ward caring for elderly male patients. During this time he needs to create a portfolio that reflects what he learns in the ward and demonstrates the clinical skills that he develops within his practice assessment tool. He will also be collecting material that he can draw on for two of the academic modules that he has to complete by the end of the academic year. One of these requires him to show his understanding of his accountability as a student nurse by reflecting on a patient he has been involved in caring for. The other asks him to demonstrate safe practice in areas of hand-washing and infection control, manual handling and moving of patients, and the basic observations of baseline physiological functioning of a patient that he has cared for. Whilst the portfolio itself will not be marked, it is a required component of his course and provides the material for monthly tutorials with his academic personal tutor. His practice supervisor will use the portfolio to assess how Mark is progressing with his practice learning objectives, and what more needs to be planned to meet his learning needs in discussion in regular supervisory meetings.

At this stage in his course, Mark will be concentrating on describing his experiences, and provide preliminary reflective accounts of these, maybe linking these to learning objectives in some way. He will be starting to develop his analytical abilities, but as the portfolio is not to be assessed in itself, he does not need to worry about the academic content. The primary purpose of this portfolio, therefore, is to collect evidence that will show that he is developing practical skills and competence, and that will give him concrete examples for his two written assignments. He chooses the 'toastrack' model to structure his portfolio because he can create separate sections headed according to what evidence he needs to collect and labels these as:

(1) practice assessment tool
    (a) proforma supplied by the university
(2) description of the ward and learning opportunities available
    (a) clinical area guide provided by the ward and practice learning facilitator, including learning opportunities available
    (b) initial discussion with practice educator/mentor/practice assessor
    (c) Mark's notes about what he wants to achieve
(3) Evidence for module one, accountability assessment
    (a) assignment guidelines for the module
    (b) copy of the NMC code of professional conduct
    (c) articles and papers on accountability
    (d) anonymous patient incidents that illustrate Mark's care delivery
(4) Evidence for module two, patient safety assessment
    (a) assignment guidelines for the module
    (b) copies of manual handling policy and procedures
    (c) evidence of attending manual handling training
    (d) articles/handouts about effective hand-washing and infection control processes
    (e) anonymous patient case material
    (f) records of care given to patients
    (g) reflective accounts of experiences in the clinical area
(5) issues to discuss with personal tutor/clinical supervisor.

Mark will primarily be using his portfolio as a convenient place to store evidence of his development. However, in choosing to use the toastrack model he provides himself with a structure that suits his immediate needs and short-term goals. The labelled sections clearly reflect where he is in his course and what he needs to achieve in the next four months. By labelling each section as he has, he has created a way of focusing on the essential material to complete his assessments. This lifts the portfolio above the shopping trolley model because it not only has a definite structure that is created to fulfil a specific purpose, but he will include his personal reflections and case material to supplement other freely available generic material such as assignment guidelines and policies. Guidance received from both his academic tutor and his clinical supervisor will help him in developing the skills of portfolio construction at this initial level. Having developed confidence in this, he will then be ready to move on to the next levels where more analytical, critical and evaluative skills need to be in evidence in the portfolio. At this stage, Mark's portfolio is not assessed for credit in his course. However, as he progresses he will be expected to demonstrate, through the original components created specifically for the portfolio, the academic and reflective skills required at higher levels of study. An example of this is outlined in Case study 6.1.

The next case study presents the decision-making taken by an experienced practitioner in planning her portfolio using the spinal column model.

Case study 6.2 Structuring a portfolio to meet the Nursing and Midwifery Council requirements for triennial registration using the 'spinal column' model.

Josie is a registered specialist community practice nurse who has been working as a health visitor for the past seven years. She is also a practice teacher who organises the practice learning for students undertaking community specialist practice routes through both undergraduate and postgraduate programmes. Her portfolio, when submitted to the NMC for auditing processes, needs to comply with requirements for periodic registration.

She also wants to use this portfolio to demonstrate her ongoing development as a practitioner for use in her annual appraisal with her manager. This will require her to analyse and evaluate her professional performance over the past year against the objectives she was set and her job description in order to come to a judgement about her work and plan for the next year. Josie has applied to her local university to undertake a Master's degree in advanced professional practice and needs to provide evidence of her work as a specialist practitioner as part of the admissions procedure. In this process she needs to be able to demonstrate how the way she practises, her skills, knowledge and experience, have prepared her for studying at this academic level, and that she has access to sufficient relevant and appropriate activities to enable her to complete her programme of study.

   She selects the 'spinal column' structure for her portfolio because it enables her to present the evidence of her achievements alongside a written reflective review of how she considers she has met them. She has chosen to label the following main sections, with each one having subsections:

(1) NMC requirements
  (a) curriculum vitae
  (b) evidence of practice standard
  (c) reflective review of evidence of CPD standard
(2) annual appraisal
  (a) appraisal record for the past year, analysis and reflective review of achievements, identification of her own developmental needs for the next year
  (b) as above for the previous year
  (c) as above for the year before that, etc.
(3) professional role development
  (a) job/role description
  (b) reflective review of how she enacts her role
  (c) identification of her own development needs arising from this analysis
(4) making a case for admission to the MSc advanced professional practice
  (a) assessment and analysis of her role against the programme's admission requirements
  (b) assessment and analysis of her own academic skills and where these may need support and development
  (c) reflective review of why she considers herself ready for this programme
  (d) assessment of how this programme will help her to develop and inform her professional practice, and what benefits this will provide to the service she works in
(5) personal development plan
  (a) reflective review of the past year's plan
  (b) incorporation of the development needs from the previous sections into her personal development plan.

   In Case study 6.2, Josie's main purpose for compiling a portfolio is to demonstrate to the Nursing and Midwifery Council that she meets the standards for continuing registration as a practitioner. However, she has structured her portfolio so that it can serve two other primary purposes as well. By selecting the spinal column model, which helps her to integrate her professional experiences with the analytical components, she is ensuring that the case she is making for each of these purposes is crystal clear to anyone who reads it. She will be analysing the evidence she is using against the standards or objectives that she needs to demonstrate and in many ways is overtly presenting the case for having achieved these to the reader. The reader has to do little work other than read the case being made in each section and match this to the evidence that Josie is presenting in support of it. She ends up by reviewing and rewriting her personal development plan for the next three years, thus giving herself clear objectives against which she can plan her next developmental activities.

Case study 6.3   Structuring a portfolio to meet assessment needs at HE level 3 (Honours) or HE level 4 (Master's) using the 'cake mix' model.

Jake is an emergency nurse practitioner working in an accident and emergency department in a large city hospital. He is midway through his Master's degree and about to submit the final module assessment in leadership and management prior to starting his dissertation. The portfolio needs to demonstrate that he has achieved the learning objectives required for the module, and in order to do this he has to show that he is applying theoretical perspectives to his practice using illustrations from his practice environment.

The 'cake mix' model suits Jake's needs best because it directs him to integrate all of the sources of his knowledge in order to demonstrate that he is working academically and in practice at Master's level. The main components of this portfolio will be Jake's reflective account(s) that analyse and critically evaluate his experiences and explore them using a range of other perspectives. It will be these components that are assessed, with the evidence simply being used to support the case he is making. The end result of this process is likely to be the creation of new knowledge, or practice theory, that results from expert practice in the field. Jake has chosen to structure his portfolio using the following sections:

(1)   contents and introduction to the portfolio, including both generic and specific objectives
(2)   the agreed learning contract
(3)   reflective review of the module (5000 words)
(4)   evidence to support the reflective review (which is referenced within the review)
(5)   the module outline including the assessment requirements.

In Case study 6.3, Jake's portfolio is clearly structured around an identified outcome that is more than the individual components that make it up. It is the process of compiling the portfolio, of the reflective work that will go into it that results in the new knowledge created. It will focus not just on what has been achieved in a concrete way, but on how Jake has arrived at his destination, providing the rationale for his decisions, and the alternatives that have informed the conclusions he has reached. Hence, the analytical and critical processes expected at Honours or Master's level will be clearly evident to the reader through the discussion that Jake creates in his reflective review. It is likely that the amount of evidence used in this portfolio will be minimal, as Jake could choose to analyse one incident, or practice development, in support of his achievement of the module learning outcomes.

Summary

- Four different models of portfolio construction within academic programmes of nursing and midwifery education have been identified by Endacott *et al.* (2004).
- These differ in their complexity, ranging from a simple collection of paper evidence gathered together, to a sophisticated primary analysis of the material that is used in evidence to support a case of achievement.
- The different structures may be used at different academic levels as the requirements for analysis and critical evaluation become more evident.

Activity

Think about the portfolio work you have done, or are being asked to do. Which type of portfolio does it most resemble? Now consider what the purpose of your portfolio is, and whether it needs to fulfil certain academic criteria in terms of reflective components, analysis, critical thinking and evaluation.

Are you using the right model?
What action would you need to take to move it from one model to another?

A portfolio structure to document professional development and accountability as a practitioner

Qualified practitioners may wish to develop their portfolio in a different way from how Josie approached it in Case study 6.2. Josie was very focused on using her short-term goals to construct her portfolio. However, other practitioners use the portfolio as a dynamic record of ongoing development in order to provide evidence of their accountability as a professional practitioner (Jasper 1999a). Portfolios of this kind are structured through outcomes, as opposed to the topic areas evident in student portfolios used for learning purposes. Jasper's (2004) model, presented in Chapter 3, relates to the way that reflective writing is used within experienced nurses' portfolios, and identifies four main components of a portfolio used in this way.

The model shows the relationship between the main components, with the dotted lines and the direction of the arrows demonstrating the strength and direction of the links. Personal development and professional development are inextricably linked; it appears that one will not happen without causing the other. Reflective writing and critical thinking appear to act as catalysts for these two types of development, with reflective writing providing the process and recognition of learning and development within the portfolio itself. The results in all cases are outcomes for clinical practice and practice development.

The four components: professional development, personal development, critical thinking and outcomes for clinical practice, can also be used as a structure for a professional portfolio and used for NMC registration purposes.

Professional development

This section of the portfolio paints a picture of the practitioner's working life, and how they have developed, changed and responded to different challenges throughout that time. Taken in isolation, this section would stand alone as a record of achievement, documenting career progression using both primary and secondary evidence. Elements of professional development include three main components:

- a continually developing knowledge base as the foundation of practice
- evidence of professional practice driven through a code of professional conduct
- evidence-based practice demonstrating considered decision-making.

Recorded in this section of the portfolio would be the practitioner's work history and/or their CV as a starting point. In addition to this the following might be added:

- their current and past job descriptions
- attendance certificates for in-service education
- academic certificates
- certificates and registration of professional qualifications
- conference or other external event attendance
- records specifically relating to the requirements of the Nursing and Midwifery Council for triennial registration
- any seminars or presentations given
- reflective reviews of any new experiences that have contributed to the practitioner's learning and development
- reflective reviews or accounts of critical incidents in practice resulting in learning or changes in practice
- records of experiences within the professional role, such as committee membership, project work, consultancy, teamworking, practice development, change management.

In short, anything can go into this section that gives the reader the picture that you want to provide of you as a professional practitioner. You may wish to focus specifically on elements of this, such as the NMC requirements that show you have constructed the portfolio for a particular purpose.

This section is essentially a 'public' section, in that it is likely that others will read or see it. It is worth bearing this in mind when deciding on the contents of the section; therefore, you may choose to view the components with an outsider's eye and consider the impression that they are giving of you as a practitioner. Just as when you put together a photograph album, you will be choosing the contents to reflect a particular viewpoint. In a photo album you may wish simply to be recording history for posterity. But you may also want to demonstrate your prowess as a photographer, or to create a particular type of history (happy, dynamic, fluid, sad) that is open for others to see. In your professional portfolio, you also have control over the type of practitioner that others see in your written evidence. The contents depend very much on what you choose to reveal about yourself.

Personal development

Whilst the professional development section tends to focus on *what* you have done as a practitioner, the personal development section is more about *how* you practise and how you have changed as a result of being a practitioner. This involves showing how you, as a person, and as part of your professional persona, develop the insight to continue to learn and develop throughout your professional career. This involves:

- using the portfolio as a developmental tool
- learning from your experiences
- utilising reflective writing as a cognitive and deliberative process
- developing your analytical and cognitive skills.

These components are a lot less tangible than those collected into the professional development section, and are less likely to be supported by 'objective' evidence. Rather, they are the kinds of things that come from within yourself, and as a result of your own written reflective activities. Rather than necessarily being open to the public gaze, this section might be entirely private, and for your eyes only.

Within this section you may therefore find:

- reflective reviews or explorations of experiences that have been difficult or uncomfortable for you
- explorations of particular patient encounters where you are dealing with your own emotional responses as opposed to patient outcomes
- reminiscences, or developing insights related to aspects of your own behaviour

- frank considerations of the role you played in an incident
- insightful examination of your own skills and abilities
- identification of your own learning and developmental needs in relation to your personal development
- records of clinical supervision from a personal viewpoint
- reflections on annual appraisal
- journal-type work that attests to development over time.

This section in a portfolio can be the most challenging and insightful, or, conversely, the least well done and most superficial. To some extent it depends on the practitioner's own willingness to engage in honest self-reflection. The success of this section in both identifying and promoting personal development rests, to some extent, upon the personal attributes and skills of the nurse identified by Atkins and Murphy (1993) as preconditions for reflective practice: self-awareness, the powers of description, critical analysis, synthesis and evaluation. In addition, the practitioner needs to feel confident in writing reflectively and willing to acknowledge the results of where that process may lead. Whilst the results of reflective activity of this sort bring tremendous rewards in terms of understanding ourselves and acknowledging our own forward journey, it can be uncomfortable along the way.

Critical thinking

The mark of a professional practitioner is that they can provide individualised care to patients on the basis of the best available evidence and their own experience and expertise. In order to do this, practitioners need to be critical thinkers who are able to draw on their knowledge, consider possible alternatives and make decisions appropriate to the particular client in front of them. Critical thinking, as facilitated through reflective writing for Jasper's (2001) practitioners, involved:

- making connections between pieces of information
- organising their thoughts in a structured way
- exploring issues from different viewpoints and theories
- taking a new perspective on issues.

The process of writing reflectively, whether using a reflective framework or not, enabled the nurses involved to find the space to explore issues in an analytical and critical way. This provides evidence in itself of the development of critical thinking. But, in addition, it illustrates the practitioner's decision-making processes, demonstrating how conclusions are arrived at having considered and rejected a range of alternatives to action.

In this section of the portfolio you may expect to see complex material, both primary and secondary, that illustrates and integrates the different ways in which professionals work. These may include:

- client case studies which have been analysed
- debates demonstrating the consideration and weighing up of evidence
- a literature review considering aspects of a topic
- analysis of clinical decisions
- critique of published papers
- analysis and self-reflection of critical decisions that have been made.

Becoming a critical thinker is not necessarily a comfortable experience as it involves taking a deliberate decision to challenge and question one's knowledge base and accepted practices. However, accountable practice requires the practitioner to be able to explain their decision-making and defend their actions. This is particularly so when those decisions and actions involve other people who trust in the professional's capabilities.

Outcomes for clinical practice

The final section of the portfolio relates to the dynamic effects of using a portfolio which result in changes in practice and practice development. The ultimate goal of this is, of course, to impact positively on patient outcomes. It is, however, notoriously difficult to 'prove' that changes to patient outcomes are related to single causes. It is also rare that a single change occurs in isolation of others going on in either the patient's journey or the care environment. This section of the portfolio provides the space for the practitioner to track and reflect upon practice development work and monitor changes to patient outcomes over time. It might include:

- the results of clinical audits demonstrating the effects of practice development
- single case studies analysing the effects of changes to practice
- evaluations of cohorts of patients
- evidence of teamworking to improve practice
- analysis of individual participation or development through planned studies, research, etc.

Summary

Each of the sections of the portfolio provides a different focus, attesting to the accountability, professional development and practice of the practitioner.

- The professional development section provides an objective overview of the practitioner's career.
- The personal development section demonstrates how they practise, exploring their own values and underpinning assumptions behind

their practice and attesting to their personal growth as a practitioner.

- The critical thinking section demonstrates their cognitive growth in analytical, critical and evaluation skills, documenting thoughtful practice in relation to their clients.
- The outcomes for clinical practice section show how the individual's own development is reflected into changing and development of practice, impacting positively on patient outcomes.

Activity

Consider the lists of evidence that you made earlier in the chapter. Try to divide them using the classification of professional development, personal development, critical thinking and outcomes for professional practice.

Does this strategy work for you?
What areas have you got an abundance of evidence for?
What areas are a bit thin and need more work?

Using this portfolio strategy provides the practitioner not only with a useful way of sorting and organising their portfolio, but also enables the practitioner to consider the balance of evidence demonstrating their professional development and practice.

Summary

- The primary function of a portfolio for a qualified practitioner is to demonstrate their accountability through evidence of their competence (or fitness) for practice.
- A portfolio structured using the four sections of professional development; personal development; critical thinking; and outcomes for professional practice enables accountability to be demonstrated.

Some strategies for portfolio construction

Whilst the basic premise of a portfolio may be to keep all your documents relating to your professional development in one place, it can actually be more proactive and exciting as a learning strategy in its own right. Any of the reflective writing strategies described in Chapter 3 can be used within your portfolio. However, I have developed some other ideas in this section that you may want to try out in your portfolio, or may be essential for particular purposes in a portfolio. These make the assumption that you will be working with your portfolio on a continuous basis so that it becomes an active and dynamic tool used regularly, as opposed to something that is compiled in retrospect. This will turn your portfolio from something compiled only for assessment, into a living and working document that provides you with an evaluative and developmental strategy for the future.

Developing a learning contract

A learning contract identifies what you are going to do, how you are going to do it, when you are going to do it by and the standard that you will achieve. It is an agreement that sets out the parameters, outcomes and courses of action that any of the parties involved in the contract sign up to. Like any other contract, it provides a standard by which something can be measured as successful or not. As it is negotiated and agreed between at least two people, it provides a clear, common understanding of what is expected. It also provides the portfolio writer with a comprehensive plan of what they want to achieve, how they can achieve it and what they need to provide to demonstrate that they have achieved it. The learning contract within a portfolio may include:

- the learning outcomes or objectives that need to be achieved
- what standard is to be achieved
- what they will do to achieve it
- what components need to be in the portfolio, including the evidence to be provided
- the criteria it will be assessed by
- the timeframe within which the portfolio is to be completed
- a plan of action for the person compiling the portfolio
- the support to be provided by others such as the practice learning facilitator, the academic staff or a mentor and the resources needed to enable the activity.

A learning contract provides the student with a certain amount of security because they have had their plans agreed in advance with the person who will be assessing them. Provided they do what they have said they will do, to the standard that is required, there should not be any problems.

Another type of learning contract can be used which is more flexible, and enables students to achieve both generic learning outcomes and ones that are specific to their own learning needs. In this way, a number of students can study the same module but achieve different learning outcomes depending upon their speciality and outcomes required. The specific learning outcomes are negotiated with the module leader and may relate to any range of activities, skills and knowledge that the student anticipates they need. This type of contract is more likely to be used in Honours or Master's level work, where students are beginning to be independent learners and working to their own interests.

Similarly, qualified practitioners may use a learning contract with their manager or clinical supervisor to devise an independent study plan within their personal development plan that will, for instance, satisfy the NMC's PREP (2004a) requirements or as a proposal for study leave within their workplace. This may be in response to certain developmental work that needs doing, such as to research the evidence to develop or change a particular practice within the working environment. Learning contracts may also be useful where an individual practitioner needs some professional or personal development to their own practice, as the agreement between the two people involved states the contractual relationship between the parties and provides a measure, in itself, of what is to be achieved and the support required.

Summary

- A learning contract is a shared agreement between at least two people about the parameters of work to be done.
- At a minimum it states what is to be achieved, how, to what standard and in what timeframe.

Using the portfolio as a workbook

Another way of using a portfolio dynamically is to make it the working document throughout a course. Jasper (1996) used the strategy of a portfolio workbook, incorporating a learning contract as the mechanism by which the students identified their learning needs and work plan throughout the whole of their nursing common foundation programme. Each week the students would be working to a given topic and predetermined learning outcomes using activities of daily living, such as eating and drinking or mobility. The students would identify:

- what they already knew about the topic
- what more they needed to know
- what skills and experience they already had
- what skills and experience they needed to gain
- how they would gain those skills and experience
- how they would demonstrate that they had achieved them; that is, the evidence that would be used.

Week by week the students built their portfolios into a comprehensive record of their achievements, demonstrating the outcomes through their activities, reflective reviews, case studies and competence assessment. By developing the portfolio as they progressed, they were able to review their progress on a weekly basis and ensure that they revisited components or outcomes that had not been completed. In this way, the students were able to build on their previous knowledge and skills, whilst at the same time spending their energies developing new knowledge and skills in order to achieve predetermined outcomes. In this study, the learning contract was key to enabling the students to maximise their study time and direct it into what was most important for them to gain in the time available. However, by the end of the programme the students had a comprehensive record of not only their achievements, and the evidence which supported them, but also a record of their development throughout the nine months. They continually built upon what had gone before, ensuring that they recognised their own professional and personal development within the framework of knowledge and skills acquisition.

This strategy is particularly useful for any learning activity that is developed over a particular timeframe, and where the portfolio needs to reflect the acquisition of knowledge and skills as well as documenting experience.

Using a learning journal

In many ways, learning journals are a variation on the portfolio workbook, but without the more prescriptive elements involved. There are many forms that a learning journal can take, from a simple descriptive record of skills and knowledge development, to a more complicated developmental journal built up over time. Techniques for incrementally revisiting and learning from critical incidents have been provided in Chapter 3. The value of a learning journal is that it focuses specifically on learning from experiences that have happened to the writer. Reflective techniques and strategies are used to explore these incidents over time, providing a developmental perspective as well as a learning experience.

Using the Nursing and Midwifery Council Code of Professional Conduct

The Nursing and Midwifery Council *Code of Professional Conduct: Standards for Conduct, Performance and Ethics* (2004b)[2] provides a useful structure for a portfolio to demonstrate accountability and competence for professional practice. The *Code* states that, as a registered nurse, midwife or specialist community public health nurse, you must:

- protect and support the health of individual patients and clients
- protect and support the health of the wider community
- act in such a way that justifies the trust and confidence the public have in you
- uphold and enhance the good reputation of the professions.

[2] The NMC *Code of Professional Conduct: Standards for Conduct, Performance and Ethics* is available at www.nmc-uk.org.

Each one of these features can be used as a section within the portfolio, with a commentary from the practitioner, together with the supporting evidence, demonstrating how that particular aspect is met. In addition, the NMC provides guidance about the specifics of accountability expected in practice, by stating the following:

'As a professional nurse or midwife, you are personally accountable for your practice. In caring for patients and clients, you must:

- *respect the patient or client as an individual*
- *obtain consent before you give any treatment or care*
- *cooperate with others in the team*
- *protect confidential information*
- *maintain your professional knowledge and competence*
- *be trustworthy*
- *act to identify and minimise risk to patients and clients.'* (NMC 2004b p. 3)

These can be incorporated throughout the four sections, or used as a feature in their own right. Suggestions for what might be included for each feature, together with the evidence that could be used, are made in Table 6.3.

Using the NMC PREP standards

The NMC PREP (NMC 2004a) practice and continuing professional development standards are established to ensure that each practitioner fulfils a minimum requirement over the previous three-year period in relation to their competence to practise. This is a very useful strategy for planning a portfolio for submission for triennial registration as a practitioner, if the portfolio is only being constructed for this purpose. It can also be used in addition to using the code of professional conduct, incorporating both elements in the same portfolio. There are two separate standards that affect a practitioner's registration: one relating to practice and one to CPD. When completing your notification to practise for triennial registration, you are signing to confirm that you:

- have worked in some capacity by virtue of your registration for a minimum of 100 days (750 hours) during the previous five years or undertaken a return to practice course (practice standard)
- undertake a minimum of 5 days (35 hours) CPD over the three-year period and record this in your personal portfolio, and make this available to the NMC for audit purposes if required to do so.

Some portfolios are audited by the NMC each year and need to provide the evidence for what has been claimed in the notification to practise. Hence, a simple portfolio structure can be used, with just two

Table 6.3 Illustration of how the NMC *Code of Professional Conduct* may be used to structure a portfolio.

Nicola is a third-year student nurse who is completing her professional development and practice module as the final part of her pre-registration programme. As the assessment for this she has to analyse her own practice and submit a portfolio demonstrating how she meets the standards outlined by the NMC. She makes the following plan as a structure for her portfolio. She needs to incorporate the elements of professional accountability within this outline.

Feature	What I understand this to mean and how I have achieved this	Examples from professional practice and evidence to support achievement
Protect and support the health of individual patients and clients Incorporate: respect for the patient or client as an individual, act to identify and minimise risk to patients and clients	My duty as a practitioner is to keep patients' welfare as paramount at all times. To do this I: Practise individualised and non-judgemental care, ensuring that all clients receive care appropriate to their needs Assess the needs of patients as individuals, including risks to their health and safety Promote equality of care, respecting differences in ethnicity, religion, gender and sexual orientation	Care plans/case studies Practice assessment document attesting competence in providing care activities Compare the care of two patients, from different age and ethnic groups for the same medical condition Examples of advocacy for patients
Protect and support the health of the wider community Incorporate: act to identify and minimise risk to patients and clients	As a nurse, I am responsible not just for looking after the sick, but for promoting health and providing patient education My actions need to incorporate infection control procedures at all times I need to assess risks to patients' and clients' health in all interactions I have with them	Records of community placement, including working with a practice nurse in vaccination and immunisation clinic, screening and health education activities Analysis of work with a health visitor in monitoring population health with specific groups; analysis of group work with young mothers

Continued

Table 6.3 *Continued*

Feature	What I understand this to mean and how I have achieved this	Examples from professional practice and evidence to support achievement
Act in such a way that justifies the trust and confidence the public have in you Incorporate: protect confidential information, be trustworthy	I need to ensure that the way I practise, talk to people and keep records respects them as private individuals I must not divulge information about other people to anyone who is not authorised to have this information I must inform people of their rights, and gain informed consent for anything that I do that involves patients and clients	Analysis of a case study used in the first section demonstrating all of these things Examples of records (anonymous) to show respectful language Critical incident analysis to discuss a personal conflict regarding a patient's rights to refuse treatment
Uphold and enhance the good reputation of the professions Incorporate: maintain professional knowledge and competence, cooperate with others in the team	I must present myself as a professional person, including the way I wear my uniform and my conduct with others I must ensure that my practice is evidence-based and justifiable to others I must work together with other people at all times and respect others' knowledge, skills and approaches to their practice	Case study to illustrate multi-professional teamworking and liaison with other agencies and demonstrating evidence-based practice

sections addressing both the practice and CPD standards. If these include both primary evidence, such as a reflective review of what has been done and achieved over the previous three years, together with the secondary evidence to support this, such as attendance certificates at study days, the portfolio will clearly demonstrate that the standards have been met.

In-depth analysis of a case study

Much of what has been said so far makes it appear that a portfolio needs to include a huge amount of paper and have separate evidence to validate every point that is being made. In fact, the skilful use of a case study can utilise a single piece of evidence, the case study itself, and cross-reference the evidence within the commentary analysing it. For instance, if the structure of the NMC *Code of Conduct* is being used, differing aspects of one case could be used as an illustration for all aspects. This could also incorporate the structure of a portfolio for professional development illustrated in the previous section, by using the headings professional development, personal development, critical thinking and outcomes for professional practice.

Summary

- A learning contract is a useful way of establishing the parameters of a portfolio, especially where it is to be externally assessed or verified.
- A portfolio workbook structure can ensure a developmental approach to skills and knowledge acquisition.
- Incremental professional development can also be recorded using learning journals.
- The NMC *Code of Professional Conduct* can be used to demonstrate professional practice.
- The NMC PREP requirements for practice and continuing professional development can be used where the portfolio is being constructed for triennial re-registration purposes.
- An analytical case study approach can be used to demonstrate multiple outcomes from one piece of evidence.

Ethical issues to be considered in portfolios

Many portfolios will be used as public documents; in other words they are likely to be seen by people other than the person who writes them. There are therefore some basic rules relating to privacy, confidentiality and ethics that portfolios need to adhere to.

Portfolios need to:

- be confidential; this means that no real names must be used when discussing cases, or places such as hospitals, practices or communities identified in the document
- involve gaining permission from others to include material about them
- use respectful language; language should be gender-free unless specifically referring to a person, be non-judgemental in terms of other people and respect individual differences
- avoid causing harm; for instance, decisions need to be made about what is included within the portfolio so that the consequences that may occur as a result are not harmful (remember that identifying incidents of misconduct and negligent behaviour may result in further action being taken)
- relate only to the development of the individual writing them; this should be the central and organising feature
- be legal.

Chapter summary

Portfolios can be used in a variety of ways to document the professional development of a practitioner. In fact, they can be seen as an essential component of professional practice, in that they provide a comprehensive record of that person's career and development over time, as well as being a dynamic strategy that can be used within the process of professional development itself. As an individualised document, the breadth of range, design and content of a portfolio, as well as the uses to which it can be put, is as varied as the number of nurses practising today. Thus, this chapter has only been able to provide some suggestions for how you may want to use and develop your portfolio depending on your needs as a practitioner.

References

Atkins, S. and Murphy, K. (1993) Reflection: a review of the literature. *Journal of Advanced Nursing*, **18**, 1188–1192.

Brown, B. (1995) *Portfolio Development and Profiling* (2nd edn). Quay Publications, Lancaster.

Endacott, R., Gray, M.A., Jasper, M.A. *et al.* (2004) Using portfolios in the assessment of learning and competence: the impact of four models. *Nurse Education in Practice*, **4**, 250–257.

Jasper, M.A. (1996) Developing a portfolio workbook for use in pre-registration education – an action research approach. In: Rolfe, G. (ed.) *Closing the Theory Practice Gap – a new paradigm for nursing*. Butterworth Heinemann, Oxford.

Jasper, M.A. (1999a) Nurses' perceptions of the value of written reflection – the genesis of grounded theory study. *Nurse Education Today*, **19**, 452–463.

Jasper, M.A. (1999b) Assessing and improving student outcomes through reflective writing. Chapter 1. In: Rust, C. (ed.) *Improving Student Learning – Improving Student Learning Outcomes*. Oxford Centre for Staff Development, Oxford.

Jasper, M. (2004) Using journals and diaries within reflective practice. Chapter 5. In: Bulman, C. and Schutz, S. (eds) *Reflective Practice in Nursing* (3rd edn), pp. 94–12. Blackwell Publishing, Oxford.

McMullan, M., Endacott, R., Gray, M.A. *et al.* (2003) Portfolios and assessment of competence: a review of the literature. *Journal of Advanced Nursing*, **41** (3), 283–294.

Nursing and Midwifery Council (2004a) *The PREP Handbook.* NMC, London.

NMC (2004b) *Code of Professional Conduct: Standards for Conduct, Performance and Ethics*. NMC, London.

7

Understanding clinical supervision: a health psychology orientated process of person-centred development

Paul Elliott

Learning objectives

Clinical supervision has been promoted as a strategy for professional development and as a way of facilitating reflective practice and clinical decision-making. As such, it is usually a relationship between at least two people (the supervisor and supervisee) and focuses on learning within the clinical role. In this chapter we will explore the underpinning nature, structure and mechanisms of clinical supervision with the intention of enabling you to understand the way it is intended to work and how to use it as a strategy in your own professional development. Clinical supervision, as a term in itself, is somewhat of a misnomer for what the process is intended to achieve. Thus, we will explore the concept of person-centred development as an alternative perspective to clinical supervision. The next sections set this in the context of health psychology. A further objective of this chapter is to challenge current thinking about clinical supervision and in so doing provide you with a more informed perspective.

By the end of this chapter you will have:

- an understanding of the principles and strategies for clinical supervision
- explored the roles of the supervisor and supervisee
- explored different models of clinical supervision
- an understanding of the processes of clinical supervision

- considered the benefits and challenges of clinical supervision
- considered the appropriateness of the term 'clinical supervision'
- considered the notion of person-centred development
- developed an understanding of how person-centred development can be facilitated.

Defining clinical supervision

Clinical supervision is a process that has been and continues to be used by many organisations and their senior practitioners towards promoting personal and professional development in their staff. Bond and Holland (1998 p. 12) define clinical supervision as: 'regular, protected time for facilitated, in-depth reflection on clinical practice'.

While this outlines the assumptions underpinning the clinical supervision relationship, the process is complicated. However, the most generally accepted definition by Faugier and Butterworth (1994) captures the essential elements as: 'an exchange between practising professionals to enable the development of professional skills'.

Essentially, clinical supervision is a process where one individual (a supervisor) facilitates one or more individuals (supervisees) in their personal and professional development through a reflective exchange (Howatson-Jones 2003 p. 37–42).

The features and underpinning philosophy of clinical supervision are:

- Each individual has the right to choose their supervisor.
- Clinical supervision should never be forced upon an individual.
- All parties within a clinical supervision setting should hold equal status, including the supervisor.
- The supervisor's role should be that of facilitator and not to dictate or decide for the supervisee.
- The clinical supervision process should be person-centred and not organisational or corporate objective centred.
- Within the clinical supervision process it must be recognised that there will be physical, psychological and social issues.
- The clinical supervision process should be underpinned by a set of mutually agreed ground rules.
- Clinical supervision should be a two-way process where all parties have the right to express, without fear of ridicule, their feelings, opinions and anxieties.
- The clinical supervision process should centre on personal and professional development in the supervisee and potentially in the supervisor.

- The clinical supervision relationship should be confidential within the context of the ground rules set.
- If written notes of clinical supervision sessions are made then copies of those notes should be made available to participants.
- Clinical supervision should occur with the consent of all parties, whether it be one-to-one or on a group basis.
- Any notes made during a clinical supervision session should remain confidential, unless otherwise agreed.

These features clearly establish clinical supervision as an interpersonal process that is focused on person-centred development for the benefit of the supervisee(s) and not necessarily the service that person is working in.

Winstanley and White (2003 p. 25) found evidence that clinical supervision was most effective if it included:

- longer sessions (around 60 minutes)
- more frequent sessions (at least monthly)
- group sessions
- sessions away from the workplace
- supervisor selection as opposed to allocation.

Activity

At this point you might like to reflect upon your own experiences of clinical supervision.

Did your experiences match your expectations?
If yes, how did they match your expectations and why do you think this was so? If no, what were the differences between your experiences and your expectations?
How did any inconsistencies make you feel about clinical supervision?

Should you choose to undertake this activity and those that follow you may find the following guide, using the 5WH cues, helpful:

Reflective key word:	Explanatory statements:
What	What, according to your interpretation, happened and how did this make you feel?
Why	Why do you feel the situation went the way it did and to what degree did your involvement affect this?
Who	Who was involved? What influence might this have had?
When	When did the situation occur and could this have influenced the outcome?
Where	Can the environment have an influence upon a situation and how it was interpreted?

How	How do you feel about what happened, what was positive and in what ways could things have gone better?

The above WH cues have been directed towards your subjective interpretation of an interaction you were involved in (or observed) and your feelings about that interaction. However, the final part of this guide is aimed at enabling you to challenge and question what you have determined about the interaction.

Who says so?	How do you know your interpretation of the situation was correct? What evidence do you have, other than your own subjective feelings, to support your interpretations? If there were others involved in the interaction would their interpretations reflect yours or could their interpretation be different?

The benefits of clinical supervision

Clinical supervision can have multiple benefits for the individual:

- a feeling of being supported and valued
- raised self-awareness
- raised self-esteem
- increased self-confidence
- facilitation of reflective thinking/practice
- greater depth of knowledge and understanding
- reduced emotional strain, stress and burnout
- personal and professional development
- a sense of personal satisfaction and achievement at work.

Many claims have been made with regard to the benefits of clinical supervision (Bowles and Young 1999 p. 958–964) including the fact that it has served to improve patient outcomes. Yet the evidence linking professional development on the part of nurses with any causal effect on improvements in patient care is thin. Winstanley and White (2003), however, suggest that the use of the Manchester Clinical Supervision Scale©, amongst other strategies, enables the efficacy of clinical supervision to be evaluated. It is suggested that effective clinical supervision, resulting in the individual benefits above, can have a knock-on effect for patients with regard to the quality of care they receive (Winstanley and White 2003).

For employers, the benefits of promoting clinical supervision are a heightened self-awareness on behalf of the supervisee, resulting in insight into their own practice and an understanding of their fallibility and accountability. For the employer, this may translate into less adverse incidents involving patients and the taking of greater professional accountability and responsibility for their practice. From a managerial point of view, clinical supervision can be manipulated to constitute a 'staff surveillance' strategy (Gilbert 2001), cloaked within the rhetoric of providing opportunities for the individual to review and modify their practice. Further, where the supervisor also acts in a line management capacity, the supervisory process can assume managerial overtones, which is contrary to the fundamental tenets of clinical supervision as a developmental process.

Terminological confusion

This leads us back to the notion of clinical supervision itself, and what appears to be terminological confusion. In comparison with the under-pinning philosophy, the title 'clinical supervision' can be argued to be wholly inappropriate and is the cause of much misunderstanding and anxiety among many individuals.

The word 'supervision', using a lay definition (*Collins English Dictionary* 2003), suggests a process of one individual directing, con-trolling or watching over others. Taken in the context of a health care setting, this can be inferred to mean within the individual's role or practice. This is clearly inappropriate in relation to the underpinning features of clinical supervision as the nature of this relationship is not one where the supervisor undertakes their role within a management context. Clearly the word 'supervision' does not carry universal meaning. With this in mind the question must be posed, why is the term 'clinical supervision' used and why has it not been discarded in favour of a more appropriate term which would reflect its actual purpose, namely that of developing, enhancing or facilitating personal and professional development?

In reflecting upon the word 'clinical', this again can lead to confu-sion as, like supervision, it does not carry universal meaning. For example, within health care the word 'clinical' may be perceived to imply involvement with patients or clients, or the undertaking of a clin-ical intervention such as surgery, bed bathing or the administration of medicines. Within a managerial setting it may be perceived as meaning 'insensitive' or 'egocentric', and within a scientific setting the word clinical may be perceived as indicating 'precise' or 'exact'. Yet none of these possible definitions adequately reflects the underpinning philosophy and features of the term.

In contrast, clinical supervision is about the supervisor facilitating and supporting the supervisees towards: challenging their own atti-tudes, values and beliefs; pushing the limits of their thinking; and questioning the status quo with regard to their own and others' work-based activities, albeit within a work, or clinical context. For example, take the attitude that a particular task or activity has always been undertaken in a certain way, so why change. The aim here would be for the supervisor to encourage the supervisee to question this approach in terms of its relevance to current and future safe working practices and whether or not such an attitude could lead to harm and damage to:

- themselves and their personal reputation
- other colleagues and their reputations
- the safety of other individuals in the working environment, such as the patients, clients and visitors
- property within the working area
- the reputation of the employer.

Another example is that of the individual who, when challenged about their failure to undertake hand hygiene between carrying out an activity like going to the toilet and then proceeding to handle food which they themselves or their colleagues or significant others may consume, responds in the following way:

> *'I am too busy trying to get things done to bother about carrying out hand hygiene and anyway why should I care? Nothing will happen to me as no one will know it was me who placed everyone at risk of contracting gastroenteritis.'*

Such attitudes can cause physical, psychological and social harm and are reflective of the 'it can't happen to me' syndrome (Elliott 2003). Further, such acts of omission, which are underpinned by an individual's attitudes, may not only constitute a breach of another's human rights (Wilkinson and Caulfield 2001) but, in the case of some employers, may lead to disciplinary action against the individual.

In essence, clinical supervision is about a supervisor facilitating a supervisee to reflect on their past, present and future behaviour and its consequences.

Summary

- Clinical supervision was introduced into professional practice during the 1920s in order to facilitate person-centred development, although its origins can be traced back to the time of Florence Nightingale (Emmerton 1999).
- It involves a relationship between two people (a supervisor and a supervisee) that is equal and focused on the needs of the supervisee.
- Clinical supervision may be undertaken on either a one-to-one basis or with multiple supervisees being facilitated by one supervisor in a group context.
- The term clinical supervision is a misnomer, in that it does not reflect the fundamental ethos of person-centred development.

Clinical supervision – a misunderstood term?

Misunderstandings of the nature of clinical supervision exist at individual, group and organisational levels. There has been inappropriate manipulation of the term 'clinical supervision', as well as the underlying concepts. Misperception of the term creates misunderstandings which may lead to a contravention of the human rights (Wilkinson and Caulfield 2001) of those receiving clinical supervision voluntarily or those forced to receive it (see Box 7.1).

Although the historical beginnings of the term 'clinical supervision' appear sketchy, one might suspect that they arose from a lack of understanding related to the incompatibility of the terms 'supervision' and 'person-centred facilitation'. In effect, the term 'clinical supervision' is a misnomer in that it implies one thing but means another. As a result, the title itself serves to flaw the whole process fundamentally because it will be subject to human perception and inference. Human perception can be defined as what each individual interprets to be true and correct following a comparison of their past experience and their interpretation of a constantly changing world around them. In essence, perception is a combination of already stored knowledge and new knowledge entering the brain through the five senses leading to the individual drawing inferences about what is happening.

Human inference can be defined as the subjective choices and decisions each individual makes about the people, environments and objects they encounter. People make inferences in order to assist them in making sense of their constantly changing world and as a means of reducing the potential for experiencing stress and anxiety.

These will undoubtedly be influenced by cognitive economic thinking (Roth and Frisby 1992) and dissonance effects (Festinger 1962). For instance, 'cognitive economy' can be seen as the individual's attempts to achieve maximum gain from minimum effort regarding the amount of thinking they have to undertake (Elliott 2003). Within the context of the term 'clinical supervision', what this means is that individuals are likely to become tunnel-visioned or context specific (Reason 1998) with regard to their understanding of clinical supervision. This, in turn, may increase the potential for misunderstanding and inappropriate manipulation of the concept by groups and organisations.

Subsequently, anything that is reliant upon such unreliable human processes is likely to severely restrict the potential positive outcomes that receiving clinical supervision can have.

It may be argued that the term can be used for purposes other than it was intended, due to the manipulative effect of the term itself; for example, individuals required to receive clinical supervision within a group or on a one-to-one basis without being given the opportunity to choose their supervisor. Yet many organisations do this because they

Box 7.1 Potential infringements of human rights in relation to clinical supervision.

Article 1 Obligations to secure rights and freedoms

Each individual has a right to receive clinical supervision if they wish. However, they also have the freedom to choose not to take clinical supervision when offered. An employee who is forced to take clinical supervision in a specific way or against their wishes might argue that their human rights have been infringed.

Article 3 Prohibition and torture

Where an individual feels they have experienced distress, pain or degrading treatment either through being forced to take clinical supervision against their wishes by an employer/manager or as a result of what they experienced during a clinical supervision session then an individual might argue that their human rights have been infringed. In addition, where an individual is forced or coerced by management to give up or make public any written notes from clinical supervision sessions which causes the individual to experience anxiety or distress then they may argue that their human rights have been infringed.

Article 8 Right to respect for private and family life

During a clinical supervision session (one-to-one or group) an individual has the right to have their privacy respected and not to be forced, coerced or socially pressured into discussing issues that may infringe upon such privacy. Where an individual considers that their privacy has not been respected within a clinical supervision session they might argue that their human rights have been infringed.

Article 9 Freedom of thought, conscience and religion

Within a clinical supervision session each individual should have the right to have and express their own thoughts, feelings and beliefs regarding topics of discussion being reflected upon. If this right is denied or restricted then the individual might argue that their human rights have been infringed.

Article 10 Freedom of expression

Within a clinical supervision session each individual has the right of expression with regard to their opinions. In addition, each individual has the right to receive appropriate information. For example, a prerequisite to supervisee and supervisor commencing a clinical supervision relationship is the establishment of ground rules where information is presented as a means of informing all parties of the boundaries within which the clinical supervision process will occur. If an individual feels they have been denied the right to express their

Continued

opinion or they feel appropriate information was not made available regarding the establishment of ground rules then they may argue that their human rights have been infringed.

Article 11 Freedom of assembly and association

If two or more employees choose to assemble on a regular basis for clinical supervision and they are denied this right by an employer/organisation then the employees might argue that their human rights have been infringed.

N.B. The above should not be perceived as being mutually exclusive but as offering a perspective.

Extracts from Wilkinson and Caulfield 2001.

believe it will do good when, in reality, imposing clinical supervision may be harmful.

Activity

What do you think the harmful effects of being forced to take part in clinical supervision might be?
What may be the consequences of not being able to choose your clinical supervisor?
You should undertake this activity before reading on.

Some of the harmful effects that might result are:

- anxiety and stress
- lack of motivation
- poor communication
- lack of mutual respect
- personality clashes
- non-attendance at clinical supervision sessions
- distrust
- hostility
- loss of self-esteem
- increased sickness and absence
- falling morale
- poor staff retention.

Whilst this list is not exclusive, it does illustrate the negative and therefore demotivational problems that may occur when practitioners do not feel valued and equal within the process of clinical supervision.

However, the imposition of clinical supervision by an organisation may also have much to do with the way they wish to be perceived; that is, as an organisation which adopts a humanistic perspective. Yet the simple act of imposition may, it could be argued, indicate anything but a humanistic approach.

Activity

At this point you might like to reflect upon the benefits of offering clinical supervision on a voluntary basis and being able to choose your supervisor.

Further, the term clinical supervision has become a jargon term integrated within common language. Thus, individuals, groups and organisations have become complacent in both their perception of the term and its application. Where organisations have imposed clinical supervision, it may become prescriptive and lead to resistance, having the opposite effect to that intended. Certainly, there is evidence to indicate that where prescriptive actions occur, the likelihood of individuals rejecting or ignoring them is significantly increased (Grilli and Lomas 1994; Reason *et al.* 1998; Lawton and Parker 1999).

Therefore the term 'clinical supervision' seems to need revision. Even if the clinical aspect were to be retained and the term 'clinical facilitation' adopted, this would not cover all eventualities. For example, applying the term 'clinical facilitation' to a management setting, a legal setting, an industrial setting or within the retail setting would be inappropriate as the term 'clinical' would lack context and would therefore be likely to cause confusion and misunderstanding. Subsequently, on the premise that the underpinning features and philosophy would be applicable to any work-based setting within health care and that every individual, irrespective of their profession, role or appointment has the right to be offered such a developmental opportunity, it would seem that a completely new term is required that will not only be universally consistent with the professions of nursing and midwifery, but within all work-based settings.

Summary

- Clinical supervision is a misnomer for the processes, concepts and underpinning features of the relationship.
- Misunderstandings may result in the individual's human rights being contravened.
- Human perception and interference, economic cognitive thinking and dissonance will all affect the ways in which clinical supervision is perceived.
- The imposition of clinical supervision and contravention of its principal features can lead to negative effects which counterbalance any positive features.

- A new term is required that articulates the processes and outcomes intended for clinical supervision more clearly.

Redefining clinical supervision

This, then, poses the question, what would constitute a more appropriate term that might carry universal meaning and be universally consistent with the underpinning philosophy? As is indicated within the title of this chapter, such a new term ought to have two principal components. First, this new term should be *person-centred*. That is, the process should be aimed at facilitating individuals towards attainment of, for example, their aspirations, enhancing their self-esteem and ultimately the individual recognising their own potential and having the confidence to become self-directed towards achieving such aims.

The second component of this new term should be orientated towards the concept of *development*. That is, where individuals are motivated towards both their personal and professional growth. For example, where nurses and midwives are concerned, the establishment, maintenance and provision of evidence within their portfolio under the Nursing and Midwifery Council's Post-registration Education and Practice requirements (NMC 2004a) could be an excellent medium for demonstrating where such personal and professional growth has occurred, is occurring and will occur.

Therefore, as an alternative to clinical supervision, the term 'person-centred development' (PCD) is offered as carrying greater universal meaning and being a more representative and humanistic reflection of the features and philosophy currently presented as clinical supervision. Figure 7.1 presents a representational perspective of the transitional process between clinical supervision and person-centred development.

Person-centred development is arguably universal in its meaning, in that the word 'person' is indicative of an individual; the word 'centred' is indicative of a focal point; and the word 'development' is indicative of growth, progress and advancement. The term 'person-centred development' is clearly more appropriate than the term 'clinical supervision' and yet there is an almost irrational persistence to continue using clinical supervision as a title for a concept for which it is clearly unsuited. In fact, it could be argued that the continued use of the term 'clinical supervision' can constitute unprofessional and unethical practice. Further, persistent use of the term could also be inferred to indicate that individuals, groups and organisations who continue to use it care little for the ethics involved and in some cases regard such ethics as secondary (Seedhouse 1998) as long as objectives are met.

Subsequently, the difficulty is likely to lie not in the development of a more appropriate alternative term but in achieving universal acceptance of a new term. Such difficulties of acceptance will have

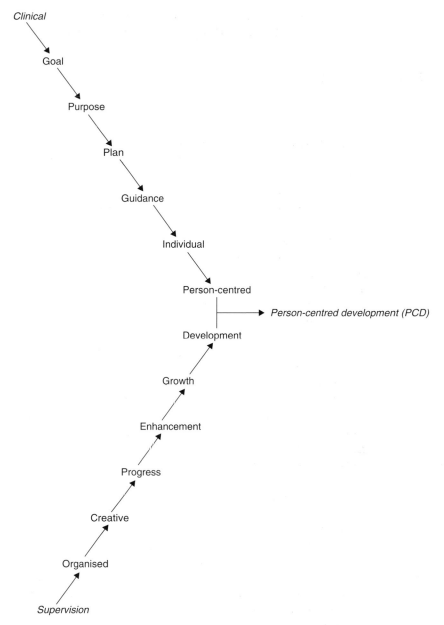

Figure 7.1 Clinical supervision in person-centred judgement: a transitional representation.

more to do with the willingness of individuals, groups and organisations to acknowledge the ethical implications and the necessity for
change.

Activity

At this point you might like to reflect upon your own feelings regarding the use
of person-centred development as an alternative term to clinical supervision.
Try to identify the reasons you think about in terms of positive and negative,
so that you can critically evaluate your own responses.

However, as with all change, whether it is for the better or worse, in
the initial instance anxiety is likely to be generated because change
requires, at least to some extent, moving from the known to the potentially unknown. Clinical supervision is a term that has been used for a
long period of time and individuals will have a preconceived understanding of what they believe the term to mean. Often though, an individual's perception of a term is not necessarily a true reflection of what
it actually should be or represents. An employer may influence their
employees' perception in accordance with how they wish a given term
to be perceived. For example, it may be that an employer will deter-

---

Box 7.2   Differences between group and one-to-one person-centred
development.

Group formatted
Several individuals agree to meet
on a regular basis with a facilitator
of their choosing, to reflect upon
issues that may serve to hinder or
enhance their personal and
professional development

In principle, there is no reason why
the facilitator cannot become an
active member of the group,
provided the group members are
comfortable with this. However,
such an approach may be viewed
as radical by some who fail to
perceive the two-way process
of development.

One-to-one formatted
Two individuals agree to meet on a
regular basis to reflect upon issues
that may serve to hinder or enhance
their personal and professional
development

In principle, one individual will fulfil
the role of facilitator, with the other
being the individual seeking to
develop themselves. However, an
ethos of person-centred development
is that development can be a two-
way process where both individuals
can have a developmental experience
as a result of each individual
bringing to the setting a unique set
of feelings, values, beliefs and ideas.

mine that clinical supervision is necessary and that the most appropriate method would be within a group format. It may be that such a decision would centre on the employer's needs and those of their employees. They may not, therefore, actively promote the idea of a one-to-one format on an equal basis and thus deny their employees the option to make an informed choice. The differences between group and individual supervision are outlined in Box 7.2.

Further, in determining that person-centred development is necessary and then restricting their employees' choice and exposure to alternatives, an employer would be contradicting the underpinning philosophy and features of the approach and may also be contravening their employees' human rights as presented in Box 7.1. However, if the employer were to present the person-centred development process as a voluntary option and within the context of an internal locus of control (Ogden 2004), although they may not capture all employees it is likely that the degree of motivation towards such a process would be enhanced. In addition, if chief executives and their senior management team were to be seen leading by example and taking person-centred development themselves, such actions might also serve to facilitate positive perceptions among their employees.

Summary

- The term clinical supervision is outdated and fails to reflect the underpinning philosophy of what it is supposed to represent.
- Clinical supervision is a term that does not carry universal meaning and is thus subject to manipulation in inappropriate ways.
- Clinical supervision should focus around two principal components: it should be person-centred and it should be developmental.
- Person-centred development (PCD) is a more humanistic and appropriate term which reflects the approach's underpinning features and philosophy and is more universally understandable with regard to its meaning and intention.
- Person-centred development should be adopted as a replacement term for clinical supervision.

The term 'person-centred development' will be used throughout the rest of this chapter instead of clinical supervision. This approach warrants a change to other, previously accepted terms, such as 'supervisor' and 'supervisee'.

Applying theories and approaches in health psychology to person-centred development

Person-centred development is a process which aims to promote personal and professional development and in so doing can have a positive effect upon an individual through reflective interaction. Such interaction can serve to facilitate physical, psychological and social well-being. Health psychology in many ways reflects the aim of person-centred development and vice versa, in that it is also concerned with the promotion of physical, psychological and social well-being in individuals. Both reflect the promotion of well-being from a lifespan perspective, thus indicating that the psychology of health and person-centred development are concerned with:

- the maintenance of health – physical, psychological and social
- the prevention and management of ill health, with prevention being of primary concern (the premise being that prevention is always preferable to cure)
- facilitating developments throughout the health care system and thus professional practice
- facilitating reflection upon health care policy and thus serving to enhance the potential for compliance (Division of Health Psychology Website 2006).

Subsequently, in consideration of the similarity between person-centred development and health psychology, this part of the chapter demonstrates the links between the two.

Origins and models

Historically, the concept of an experienced individual offering guidance to someone less experienced within nursing can be traced back to the time of Florence Nightingale (Emmerton 1999). From the mid-1920s this concept was applied within the field of psychotherapy. However, it was not until the late 1980s that person-centred development, in the inappropriate guise of clinical supervision, was presented and applied in the form of professional development (Winstanley and White 2003). Subsequently, a variety of clinical supervision models have been developed, some of which are presented within Table 7.1.

Activity

Before reading on, think about how you feel about each of the models outlined in Table 7.1.

Which would you prefer to be applied to your person-centred development sessions and why?

The developmental (Leddick 1994), practice-centred (Sloan and Watson 2002) and the friendship (Smith 2000) models adopt a humanistic

Table 7.1 Examples and overview of clinical supervision models.

Model type	Descriptive overview
Developmental	Underpinning this model is the premise that individuals are continually growing, the aim being to identify new areas of growth within the context of lifelong learning.
Integrated	Within the context of this model the supervisor can take the role of teacher in directly lecturing, instructing and informing the supervisee towards identifying their needs.
Orientation-specific	A premise of this model is that during the initial stages of the relationship supervisor and supervisee will observe each other for signs of expertise and weakness leading to each party attributing influence and authority over the other. (Extracts from Leddick 1994)
Practice-centred	This model would seem to include within its framework education, support, objective setting and practice analysis. It is similar to Proctor's three-function interactive model but substitutes the above for Proctor's normative, formative and restorative aspects. (Extracts from Sloan and Watson 2002)
Friendship	It would seem that underpinning this model is the premise that individuals involved in the relationship will gain some good from the experience. All parties are useful to each other but this usefulness can change over time and once the association is fulfilled it can be easily dissolved. Such an approach can be seen to exist within the context of the person-centred development relationship where it is underpinned by the development and regular review of a contract in the guise of ground rules. (Extracts from Smith 2000)

These should not be seen as being mutually exclusive where types of clinical supervision model are concerned.

perspective, to some degree, in that they reflect some aspects of the person-centred development approach and process.

However, the practice-centred model also indicates a managerial classification and the incorporation of counselling skills, neither of which are aspects of the person-centred development process. The person-centred development process is not intended to include management in any form as this implies a biomedical approach (Ogden 2004). It is without doubt inappropriate for an individual to be facilitated in their person-centred development by a line manager or any individual holding a management position if that manager is likely to be in a position where they may have a conflict of interest. For example, if an individual's person-centred development facilitator was also their line manager and they needed to instigate disciplinary action against the individual this would constitute a conflict of interest at a professional, moral and ethical level, and may well have implications under the Nursing and Midwifery Council *Code of Professional Conduct* (NMC 2004b). Incorporating counselling skills as part of the person-centred facilitator's role could potentially constitute dangerous practice unless the facilitator had previously undertaken specialist and recognised counselling education and training. For example, nurses and midwives do not receive specific and externally recognised education and training in counselling during pre-registration education.

Yet many within the professions of nursing and midwifery hold dissonance-based beliefs (Festinger 1962) that they can counsel and that their nursing and midwifery qualification qualifies them to do so. Thus, when a nurse or midwife takes on the role of a person-centred development facilitator their dissonance-based belief is likely to be reinforced by such models that include reference to counselling, when in reality they are neither qualified nor competent to counsel anyone, and certainly not within a person-centred development relationship. Counselling is a skilled profession in its own right and for any model to include or imply that counselling is a part of the person-centred development facilitator's role is promoting potentially dangerous practice which could result in disastrous outcomes. The integrated and orientation-specific models (Leddick 1994) may not be seen to reflect the process and are biomedical (Ogden 2004) in their approach. Box 7.3 outlines the biomedical approach applied to person-centred development.

However, all the models presented within Table 7.1 have one thing in common. They fail to account for or reflect adequately a biopsychosocial approach (Engle 1980; Ogden 2004) to the person-centred development process, in that consideration must always be given to physical, psychological and social factors.

Summary

- Models of clinical supervision have their origins in psychotherapy.
- A number of models of clinical supervision exist, each having a different focus to the approach.
- None of the models adequately reflect a biopsychosocial approach.

Using the biopsychosocial approach

Features of the biopsychosocial approach are given in Table 7.2.

The notion that underpins the biopsychosocial approach centres around the need for facilitators to have an understanding that integral to the person-centred development process and during person-centred development sessions there will always be physical, psychological and social factors impacting on those present. Thus, the outcome of any person-centred development session will, to a great extent, be deter-

---

Box 7.3 The biomedical model applied to person-centred development.

The origins of a biomedical approach emanate from a model of health care practice going back some 2000 years, a synopsis of which is set out within Ogden (2004). The features below have been adapted from this model to reflect a perspective which is neither person-centred nor consistent with the features underpinning PCD.

(1) Individuals are denied the right to choose their facilitator (supervisor).

(2) Person-centred development should be imposed upon a workforce or body of individuals without prior consultation with those individuals.

(3) Person-centred development can include a management component and thus the role of facilitator (supervisor) can be performed by an individual's line manager.

(4) Facilitators (supervisors) are present to lecture and instruct as opposed to facilitate.

(5) Each individual within the person-centred development setting should seek to influence and exert authority over others present.

(6) Person-centred development is not about individual growth and facilitation but should be implemented as a means of achieving the employer's needs and objectives.

(7) Inappropriate manipulation of the person-centred development philosophy is acceptable and carries ethical or human rights implications.

(8) Cognitively economic and dissonance-based thinking among individuals regarding person-centred development should be encouraged as a means of exercising control through maintaining anxiety, stress and confusion leading to successful manipulation of the person-centred development philosophy.

(9) Use of the term clinical supervision, which is a misnomer and therefore a medium though which individuals can be misinformed, is acceptable despite the ethical and human rights issues.

(10) The application of an external locus of control within the person-centred development process is acceptable.

The above should not be seen as being mutually exclusive with regard to linking person-centred development and a biomedical approach.

---

mined by the facilitator's ability to understand, integrate and apply these factors towards the achievement of positive outcomes. An example of each factor is:

(1) Physical: in the case of *fatigue,* having an understanding that this may impact upon both the amount and quality of communication that occurs. An individual who is fatigued is likely to be more susceptible to misinterpretation regarding what is being

Table 7.2 The biopsychosocial model applied to person-centred development.

The biopsychosocial model originates from the work of Engle (1980). The features below have been adapted from this model, a synopsis of which is set out by Ogden (2004) to reflect a perspective that is consistent with the underpinning philosophy of person-centred development. *Factors which can inform and impact upon the person-centred development relationship*:

Physical aspects	Psychological aspects	Social aspects

• The environment:
  temperature
  ventilation
  lighting
• Time of day
• Workload
• Physical fatigue
• Absence of hunger
  and thirst
• Comfort:
  seating
  positioning
  body space
• Flexible working
• Linking PCD sessions
  to duty rotas
• Identification of
  dedicated time for
  PCD to occur
	• Mood
	• Degree of stress/anxiety
	• Motivation
	• Communication:
	  verbal
	  non-verbal
	• Sense of personal safety
	• Attitudes
	• Freedom of choice
	• Sense of acceptance
	• Sense of belonging
	• Promotion of self-esteem
	• Freedom from ridicule
	• Feeling valued
	• Past experience
		• Maintenance of dignity
		• Confidentiality
		• Establishment of agreed
		  ground rules
		• Sense of equality
		• Facilitation not dictation
		• Self-expression
		• Receiving appropriate
		  information
		• Personal gain
		• Provision of education
		  aimed at defining
		  person-centred
		  development and
		  dissemination of
		  information
		  to all employees

Individuals should be offered PCD but not forced to take it. They should be given the facts and allowed to make an informed decision but not coerced in any way.

Individuals should be allowed to choose their PCD facilitator and where this may not be possible, in the case of a new member of staff arriving within the work environment, they should be supported if they would prefer not to have the PCD facilitator allocated to them.

The above should not be seen as being mutually exclusive.

communicated, whether this is verbal or non-verbal in nature. Therefore, a good facilitator will be adequately prepared to defuse any situation of misinterpretation should it occur.

(2) Psychological: in the case of *freedom of choice*, having an understanding of the consequences that may result from an individual being forced to have person-centred development and/or being unable to choose their own facilitator and how this will be likely to have an impact upon that person's degree of motivation towards attending person-centred development sessions. Therefore, a good facilitator will be prepared to acknowledge that they may not be the most appropriate person and should offer the recipient of person-centred development the opportunity to choose another facilitator. Also, it is important to present the pos-

itive aspects of receiving person-centred development from the perspective, 'what's in it for me?' Using this approach can be a useful psychological strategy when attempting to motivate an individual towards doing something that initially they may not want to do.

(3) Social: in the case of establishing *agreed ground rules*, having an understanding of the need to do this for all concerned and that the implications of not doing so may lead to conflict and distrust in the future. Establishing mutually agreed ground rules is vital for the smooth progression of future person-centred sessions. Having a set of ground rules provides all parties with the boundaries for the sessions and the nature of the relationship. A good facilitator will ensure that such ground rules are established during the initial part of the first person-centred development session.

Activity

Spend some time thinking about the biomedical and biopsychosocial models. Looking at the underpinning philosophy and features, which do you feel would be more appropriate to person-centred development?

When you have done this, give some thought to why you feel the way you do.

As you will probably have determined, a biopsychosocial approach to person-centred development is vastly more appropriate than a biomedical approach because not only does the biomedical approach fail to reflect the underpinning philosophy of person-centred development, but also only primarily accounts for the physical factors that will be inherent within any person-centred development session. In addition, the models presented in Table 7.1, as a result of their failure to reflect a truly biopsychosocial approach to person-centred development, are questionable in terms of their validity and reliability in setting out to promote the maintenance of health, the prevention and management of ill health, the facilitation of developments throughout the health care system, or to facilitate reflection upon health care policy.

In contrast, it is arguable that a biopsychosocial approach to person-centred development will encompass all these and indicate that a health psychological perspective underpinning person-centred development will be far more holistic and thus more appropriate in terms of personal and professional development. Other theories and approaches within health psychology that will serve to reinforce this premise are presented within Figure 7.2, some of which have already been alluded to.

Within the context of person-centred development, locus of control (Rotter 1975: Wallston and Wallston 1982) has two dimensions. When

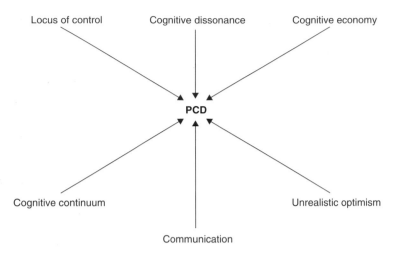

The terms identified above are drawn from Ogden (2004) and positioned to represent a link with PCD.
The above should not be seen as being mutually exclusive with regard to theories and approaches within health psychology that may be applicable to PCD.

Figure 7.2 Theories and approaches within health psychology applicable to person-centred development.

applied to the concept of person-centred development an internal locus of control would be indicative of an individual being offered choices, provided with appropriate information and being actively involved within their person-centred development process. In contrast, an external locus of control as applied to person-centred development would be indicative of an individual having person-centred development forced upon them, having their facilitator chosen for them, being provided with incorrect or manipulated information and denied any involvement in how their person-centred development process will develop and move forward.

Clearly, the adoption of an internal locus of control is consistent with the features of person-centred development and a biopsychosocial approach in that, for example, it acknowledges all parties within the person-centred development process as having equal status as well as having physical, psychological and social needs. It is therefore well suited as a theory to underpin the link between health psychology and the person-centred development process. In contrast, the adoption of an external locus of control with regard to person-centred development is clearly inappropriate.

Cognitive dissonance (Festinger 1962) is related to the premise that although an individual may believe they are rational and thinking or behaving in a rational way, they are in fact rationalising their thoughts and/or behaviour in order to make them consistent with what they perceive to be socially, morally, professionally or ethically acceptable.

However, such perceptions are not necessarily guaranteed to be a true reflection of reality and for the most part are based upon an individual's expectations. Therefore, dissonance effects may be defined as the excuses an individual generates to justify what thinking or behaviours they have previously carried out, are currently carrying out or want to carry out in the future. Such excuses will then serve to reduce any stress, anxiety or psychological conflict generated in the individual.

Taken within the context of person-centred development, such rationalisations can be influenced by:

- the environment within which person-centred development takes place
- the culture, gender and age of others present at the person-centred development session
- each individual's understanding of person-centred development and its purpose
- the attitude towards person-centred development that each individual holds
- the individual's understanding of person-centred development
- what an employer has led an individual to believe about person-centred development
- what their peers have told the individual about person-centred development
- the individual's own past experience of person-centred development
- fear of retribution and consequences to self
- the absence of individual choice.

For example, an individual may rationalise that person-centred development is of little value to their particular situation because:

- they only work part time
- they only work to supplement their partner's primary income
- they are far too busy to worry about such things
- they are, in the case of a nurse or midwife, too busy meeting their patients'/clients' needs to bother with person-centred development
- they do not understand the concept and thus reject person-centred development as being of little value out of dissonance-based fear of the unknown.

However, although individuals may consider these to be rational reasons for rejecting person-centred development, it does not hold that what is rationalised is automatically rational. Such irrational rationalisation can affect the uptake of person-centred development, impact upon attendance at person-centred development sessions and serve to disrupt the interactions that occur during these sessions. Subsequently, facilitators of person-centred development sessions must be alert to such rationalisations and in recognising them, act to facilitate the individual in reflecting on, and dealing with, their perceptions.

Cognitive economy (Roth and Frisby 1992) can be linked closely with dissonance effects in that they complement each other in producing negative and unrealistic perceptions regarding person-centred development. Furthermore, they can combine to influence interactions that occur within person-centred development sessions. For example, an individual's cognitive economic perspective towards person-centred development as a result of their poor understanding of what it is intended to provide, can lead to reduced levels of communication and inappropriate verbalisations and body language, the appearance of prejudice and stereotyping, misunderstandings and misinterpretation, feelings of distrust and isolation within person-centred development sessions, and an overall lack of personal and professional development which is contrary to the essence of person-centred development. Individuals who lack sufficient information and understanding of person-centred development will become cognitively economic (tunnel-visioned) in their perspective and will tend to fill in any gaps with intuitive based perspectives which may be unreliable and are usually incorrect. In other words, what they do not know they will make up as they go along. Facilitators of person-centred development need to be aware of the consequences of economic cognitive thinking as it can serve to disrupt person-centred development sessions.

The cognitive continuum that is presented within Figure 7.3 has been drawn from the work of Hamm (1984) and adapted to reflect levels of communication within the person-centred development process.

The continuum has six levels and no one level should be seen to exist in isolation. Within the person-centred development session, for communication to occur at one level in isolation is likely to promote dissonance effects and cognitively economic perspectives. Applying levels one and two in isolation without the inclusion of the other levels may lead to misinterpretation and misunderstanding. Just because a given issue or finding is research or evidence-based it does not automatically imply that it is appropriate for application within the real world of health care practice. In isolation, research and evidence are only validated by the information provided. Subsequently, if appropriate personal and professional development is to occur as a result of person-centred development then decision-making and problem-solving through communication must involve all levels of the continuum. Within the person-centred development process accurate and effective communication is vital and without such, person-centred development will be destined to failure, leading to potential physical distress, psychological harm and social discontent among individuals involved. Employers and person-centred development facilitators must be acutely aware of this and that the success or failure of person-centred

(1) = Research-based interaction:
Communication within the PCD session uses research evidence to facilitate personal and professional development.

(2) = Evidence-based interaction:
Communication within the PCD session applies clinical evidence towards the facilitation of personal and professional development.

(3) = Reflection-based interaction:
Communication within the PCD uses to one degree or another reflective thinking towards the facilitation of personal and professional development.

(4) = System-aided interaction:
Communication within the PCD session can be facilitated through the use of technology towards facilitating personal and professional development.

(5) = Peer group based interaction:
Communication within the PCD session is facilitated through the discussion that occurs between those present as a means of facilitating personal and professional development.

(6) = Intuition-based interaction:
Communication within the PCD session is facilitated through intuitive thinking (gut feeling) as a means of facilitating personal and professional development.

Adapted From Hamm 1984 and Elliott 2003.

Figure 7.3 The cognitive continuum related to person-centred development.

Table 7.3 Examples of verbal and non-verbal forms of communication which may impact on person-centred development sessions.

Verbal	Non-verbal
• Feminine and masculine voices	• Facial expression
• Tones of voice	• Degree of eye contact
• Accents and dialects	• Line of sight when not making eye contact
• Language used	• Hand gestures
• Cultural inflections	• Position and movement of arms and legs
• Rate of speech	• Proximity to others (body space)
• Inappropriate/repetitive apologising or the sorry syndrome	• Type and era of clothing worn
• Use of jargon	• Hair style and length
	• Type and location of jewellery worn
	• Attractiveness to others

development can come from two communication dimensions, verbal and non-verbal (see Table 7.3).

In continuing to reflect upon the link between health psychology and person-centred development, unrealistic optimism (Weinstein 1984) can also serve to impact upon an individual's personal and professional development. For example, where an individual has no personal experience of person-centred development they may view it from a 'perceived risk to themselves' perspective and thus begin to develop unrealistic beliefs about the nature of person-centred development. Both of these can be related directly to the establishment of dissonance effects, leading to cognitive economic thinking, resulting in functioning at levels five and six of the cognitive continuum. These, when working together, serve to reflect a biomedical approach. Subsequently, employers and facilitators must develop an awareness of the consequences that unrealistic optimism can have upon an individual's perception of person-centred development.

This further highlights the need for a biopsychosocial approach towards the implementation of person-centred development. Certainly, when attempting to promote the idea of person-centred development, whether it be in the initial instance or on an ongoing basis, an employer and facilitators must give consideration to how individuals will interpret what they are told and presented with, whilst recognising that each individual may do this in a uniquely different way.

Activity

Reflect back upon what you have read and consider the advantages and disadvantages of underpinning person-centred development with theories and approaches in health psychology.

Summary

- Although there are many models of clinical supervision the majority do not reflect a biopsychosocial approach to the concept of person-centred development.
- Direct links can be shown to exist between health psychology and person-centred development.
- Health psychology can provide a theoretical framework from which person-centred development can function.
- Adopting a biomedical approach to person-centred development constitutes professional, ethical, moral and human rights issues.
- Use of the term 'clinical supervision' is no longer appropriate and should cease as it fails to reflect the underpinning philosophy.
- Continued use of the term clinical supervision constitutes a disregard for the morality, ethics and human rights where personal and professional development is concerned.
- Person-centred development (PCD) is a more appropriate term and reflects the underpinning philosophy and a biopsychosocial approach; it does not present the same professional, ethical, moral and human rights issues that clinical supervision does.
- Person-centred development should therefore replace the term 'clinical supervision' on a universal basis.

Roles within the person-centred development process

Although roles with the person-centred development process can be defined as 'facilitator' and 'recipient' there should be no hierarchical structure. The facilitator does not operate within a person-centred development session to control or dictate. Rather, they are there to smooth the progress of the session and should be undertaking the role of facilitator by consent of those receiving person-centred development. The role of the facilitator includes:

- an educative function
- an evaluative function
- a support function
- facilitation of the relationship
- facilitation of the process of person-centred development
- facilitation of critical analysis and reflection
- empathetic support
- change agent
- transmission of knowledge
- maintaining the ground rules agreed
- maintaining confidentiality
- conducting sessions in an ethical and respectful way
- using non-discriminatory language.

All of these are undertaken within the precept of facilitating the recipient of person-centred development to explore and fulfil their own developmental needs. Whilst these needs are subject to negotiation between the facilitator and recipient(s) of person-centred development, the facilitator's own personal needs may also be part of the relationship. Fowler (1995) found that students' perceptions are that a good facilitator:

- forms a relaxed and supportive relationship
- has relevant knowledge and skills
- can assess learning needs, supervise and evaluate learning
- is aware of the pressures and demands of the course and the students' previous experience
- demonstrates effort in putting themselves out to help the students.

This is in direct contrast to the facilitator who has their own agenda for a meeting, and is also in a position of power over the recipients of person-centred development.

The role of the recipient is to interact with the facilitator and any others present, with the aim of enhancing personal and professional development in order to develop their own and others' human interaction skills and safe functioning within the workplace. In addition, all those present within person-centred development sessions, irrespective of their designated roles, should act as if in a partnership where all are of equal status regardless of their position, appointment or standing within an organisation. On occasions, it may well be that the roles of facilitator and recipient will be interchangeable because the person-centred development process is two-way in nature where, for example, the facilitator may find themselves in a position where the recipient is serving to enhance their personal and professional development. The recipient has certain responsibilities within the relationship and process:

• to be clear about the focus of developmental activity
• to agree the ground rules of the relationship
• to participate willingly in the process
• to respect the facilitator
• to engage in critical reflection.

The recipient's role may also include making a record of the interaction, keeping notes, or engaging in further activity as a result of the meeting. Following through on agreed outcomes is as much a part of the process of person-centred development as the interaction between facilitator and recipient itself, as it is this that leads to observable change and development in practice.

In essence, roles, in this case facilitator and recipient, are subjective labels we apply in order to help us make sense of an event, a situation, an experience or the world around us, but they are only labels and can be inappropriate, misleading and unsafe, as has been shown to be the case regarding the term 'clinical supervision'. However, even more positive labels such as 'facilitator' and recipient are still labels and as such all labels should never be perceived as being absolutes. Rather they should be highly flexible within the underpinning concepts of the process within which they exist, in this case person-centred development. Further, if labels such as person-centred development, facilitator or recipient are to be used then they should also be seen to carry universal meaning in accordance with what it is they are intended to represent, in this case a process of personal and professional development.

Other roles related to the person-centred development process

The role of a *person-centred development facilitator* can be contrasted with those of a *mentor* and *preceptor* in that they are all roles where the facilitation of personal and professional development is paramount.

Traditionally, the role of mentor has been viewed as relating to the facilitation of pre-registration health care professional students and exists within the bounds and confines of a given clinical placement or programme of pre-registration health care education. Mentors, as opposed to facilitators of person-centred development, usually have a supervisory and assessment component to their role, and are involved in enabling the development of the student as a safe and competent practitioner. The nature of the mentor's role is therefore significantly different to that of a person-centred development facilitator, who may, or may not, be involved with the clinical practice aspects of the recipient's work. Meary (2000) suggests that the mentor's role includes three support systems:

- educative: involving assessment and offering feedback to students as well as facilitating their learning
- psychological support: being a friend, advisor and motivator
- managerial: suggesting liaison with appropriate staff to achieve learning opportunities and ensuring the learning environment is safe. (Meary 2000 adapted from Maddison 2004).

The mentoring role is always likely to be one of unequal status, where a more experienced practitioner supervises a less experienced colleague. Whilst elements of person-centred development may take place within this, it is difficult to achieve the underpinning fundamental features of person-centred development where this imbalance occurs.

Preceptorship is perceived as being related to the facilitation of newly qualified practitioners and those practitioners entering a new area of practice. However, the preceptorship role is generally seen as being short term, usually counted in months, until the practitioner is deemed competent and/or feels confident to function safely within a given area of practice. Person-centred development, however, is intended to facilitate individuals on a lifespan basis and within the context of health care from point of entry to an individual's chosen profession or appointment until retirement.

In consideration of this it would seem that in comparison to the lifespan nature of person-centred development both the mentor and preceptor roles are limited in that their time span is predetermined. Yet it can be argued that their purpose and intent is similar to that of a facilitator of person-centred development. This then poses the question, if all three have the same underpinning intent why do we have person-centred development facilitators, mentors and preceptors? It is essentially the context and outcomes intended within these roles that differentiates them, whilst accepting that professional and personal development is the ultimate focus of all three relationships. Whatever the reason, each of the roles involves learning, assessment intended to facilitate development and reflection both in and on work-based activities.

Using person-centred development as a strategy for personal and professional development

The use of person-centred development as a strategy for personal and professional development has to be viewed within the context of human behaviour modification which always has been and continues to be difficult to achieve. A clear example of where such behaviour modification has been generally unsuccessful is hand hygiene among those involved in the provision of health care. Despite significant efforts on the part of many health care providers and centres of higher education, poor or inadequate hand hygiene continues to generate cause for concern (Elliott 1996; Thomas *et al.* 2005) with regard to the transmission of health care acquired infection. If person-centred development, as a facilitator of such behaviour modification, is to have any kind of success it must be viewed in the wider context as one of a number of strategies aimed at effecting some level of behavioural modification relevant to the enhancement of safe working practices. The success of person-centred development in isolation may serve to achieve only limited behavioural modification and it should not be perceived as an all-consuming process that will put everything right.

However, when combined with other developmental strategies such as those listed below, the person-centred development process can be viewed as one of a range of developmental activities all focused on facilitating lifelong learning and personal and professional development:

- PREP
- maintaining a personal reflective journal
- an open, caring, sharing approach by employers where information provision is concerned
- the development and maintenance of a personal portfolio
- education and training being readily available
- the establishment of a questioning culture where the words, *who; what; when; where; how; why and who says so* become synonymous with corporate identity
- the availability of person-centred development being made highly visible
- corporate objectives that serve to reflect the value of person-centred development and not vice versa
- those at the top of an organisation being seen to be leading by example where the taking of person-centred development is concerned.

Within an organisation, person-centred development as one strategy among others can, however, become the lynchpin from which all other strategies emanate. In essence, person-centred development is an essential component of any organisation where that organisation claims to be person-centred.

Chapter summary

This chapter has attempted to present a new way of thinking with regard to your personal and professional development, and where person-centred development (or as it should no longer be known, 'clinical supervision') fits within this. It has raised issues that might be classed as controversial and that challenge the status quo. No apology is made for this as the intention has been to generate discussion, debate and critical reflection on your part.

Activity

Ask yourself the following question:

What have I learnt from reading this chapter and undertaking the activities? Make a list of what you decide and compare it with the content of the chapter. In doing this it will help to consolidate what you have learnt.

References

Collins (2003) *Collins English Dictionary.* Harper Collins, Glasgow.

Bond, M. and Holland, S. (1998) *Skills of Clinical Supervision for Nurses.* Open University, Buckingham.

Bowles, N. and Young, C. (1999) An evaluative study of clinical supervision based on Proctor's three-function interactive model. *Journal of Advanced Nursing,* **30** (4), 958–964.

Division of Health Psychology (2006) *What is Health Psychology?* Available online at: http://www.health-psychology.org.uk/menuItems/what_is_health_psychology.php (accessed February 2006).

Elliott, P. (1996) Hand-washing practice in nurse education. *Professional Nurse,* **11** (6), 357–360.

Elliott, P. (2003) Recognising the psychosocial issues involved in hand hygiene. *The Journal of the Royal Society for the Promotion of Health,* **123** (2), 88–94.

Emmerton, A. (1999) Address given at Florence Nightingale memorial service. Westminster Abbey, London.

Engle, G.L. (1980) The clinical application of the biopsychosocial model. *American Journal of Psychiatry,* **137**, 525–544.

Faugier, J. and Butterworth, T. (1994) *Clinical Supervision: a Position Paper.* University of Manchester, Manchester.

Festinger, L. (1962) Cognitive dissonance. *Scientific American,* **207**, 93–102.

Fowler, J. (1995) Nurses' perceptions of the elements of good supervision. *Nursing Times*, **91** (22), 33–37.

Gilbert, T. (2001) Reflective practice and clinical supervision: meticulous rituals of the confessional. *Journal of Advanced Nursing*, **36** (2), 199–205.

Grilli, R. and Lomas, J. (1994) Evaluating the message: the relationship between compliance rate and the subject of a practice guideline. *Medical Care*, **32** (3), 202–213.

Hamm, R.M. (1984) Clinical intuition and clinical analysis: expertise and the cognitive continuum. In: Dowie, J. and Elstein, A. (eds) (1996), *Professional Judgement – a Reader in Clinical Decision-making.* Cambridge University Press, Cambridge.

Howatson-Jones, I.L. (2003) Difficulties in clinical supervision and lifelong Learning. *Nursing Standard*, **17** (37), 37–41.

Jasper, M. (2003) *Beginning Reflective Practice.* Nelson Thornes, Cheltenham.

Lawton, R. and Parker, D. (1999) Procedures and the professional: the case of the British NHS. *Social Science and Medicine*, 48, 353–361.

Leddick, G.R. (1994) Models of clinical supervision. *ERIC Digest.* Available online at: http://www.ericdigests.org/1995-1/models.htm (accessed February 2006).

Nursing and Midwifery Council (NMC) (2004a) *The PREP Handbook.* NMC, London.

Nursing and Midwifery Council (2004b) *Code of Professional Conduct: Standards for Conduct, Performance and Ethics.* NMC, London.

Ogden, J. (2004) *Health Psychology – a Textbook* (3rd edn). Open University Press/McGraw-Hill, Maidenhead.

Reason, J. (1998) *Human Error.* Cambridge University Press, Cambridge.

Reason, J., Parker, D. and Lawton, R. (1998) Organisational controls and safety: the varieties of rule related behaviour. *Journal of Occupational and Organisational Psychology*, **71**, 289–304.

Roth, I. and Frisby, J.P. (1992) *Perception and Representation – a Cognitive Approach.* Open University Press, Milton Keynes.

Rotter, J. (1975) Some problems and misconceptions related to the construct of internal versus external control of reinforcement. *Journal of Clinical Psychology*, **43**, 56–67.

Seedhouse, D. (1998) *Ethics: the Heart of Health Care* (2nd edn). John Wiley and Sons, Chichester.

Sloan, G. and Watson, H. (2002) Clinical supervision models for nursing: structure, research and limitations. *Nursing Standard*, **17** (4), 41–46.

Smith, G. (2000) *Friendship within Clinical Supervision: a Model for the NHS.* Presentation for launch of National Nursing Strategy for Wales: Realising the Potential (September).

Thomas, M., Gillespie, W., Krauss, J. *et al.* (2005) Focus group data as a tool in assessing effectiveness of a hand hygiene campaign. *American Journal of Infection Control*, **33** (6), 368–373.

Wallston, K.A. and Wallston, B.S. (1982) Who is responsible for your health? The construct of health locus of control. In: Sanders, G.S. and Suls, J. (eds) *Social Psychology of Health and Illness.* Erlbaum, Hillsdale.

Weinstein, N. (1984) Why it won't happen to me: perceptions of risk factors and susceptibility. *Health Psychology*, **3**, 431–457.

Wilkinson, R. and Caulfield, H. (2001) *The Human Rights Act – a Practical Guide for Nurses.* Whurr, London.

Winstanley, J. and White, E. (2003) Clinical supervision models, measures and best practice. *Nurse Researcher*, **10** (4), 7–38.

Practising as a professional

Learning objectives

This chapter explores the implications of having a professional registration for professional practice in terms of the concepts that underpin that practice as an everyday activity. Many of the standards for practice fall within the remit of the Nursing and Midwifery Council, who impose duties and responsibilities upon practitioners in return for a licence to practise independently. Nurses can identify their own professional development needs by exploring the parameters of professional practice and identifying and planning to meet their learning and developmental needs.

By the end of this chapter you will have:

- considered your roles and responsibilities as a professional practitioner
- framed your own practice within the Nursing and Midwifery Council *Code of Professional Conduct*
- an understanding of the notion of professional accountability
- explored the scope of professional practice, competence and fitness to practise
- considered the implications of confidentiality, informed consent, the Data Protection Act 1998 and the Freedom of Information Act 2000
- framed your own professional development within the boundaries of professional practice.

Activity

Take a few minutes to write down what it means to you to be a registered or student practitioner.

What guides your practice?
How autonomous are you as a practitioner?
How do you determine how to behave as a professional?
How do you assess the standards and quality of your practice?
How do you know what you should be achieving as a professional?

Introduction

This chapter asks you to consider your own practice against published standards from the NMC, from pertinent Governmental guidance, and from legal standards. No professional can practise outside the legal framework that licenses them to practise, or outside the code of professional conduct imposed by their professional body when they are admitted to the professional register.

These parameters for practice provide excellent guidance for a practitioner's professional development, as they provide a starting point for analysing practice, identifying good practice and diagnosing learning needs and where practice needs to be updated in order to meet the standards of practice required. This chapter enables you to do this using the self-assessment activities throughout. Each section will provide a summary of the standard of practice expected. You will be encouraged to:

- reflect on your own practice
- consider your understanding of the guidance presented
- assess your current practice
- identify good practice
- identify your learning and professional development needs
- identify changes to practice that might be required.

This could be done as part of constructing your professional portfolio, as you will be providing the evidence to show how your practice complies with the code of professional conduct, and how your practice has developed as a result.

What is 'professional practice'?

At a fundamental level, professional practice is about what you do as a result of being registered with a professional body: the Nursing and Midwifery Council. On becoming a registered practitioner you are expected to take on the features of what that profession is. These expectations come from a variety of sources:

- the professional body itself, as it lays down the *Code of Professional Conduct: Standards for conduct, performance and ethics*, that all registrants must adhere to during their practice
- the legal system, in that the profession is regulated by law
- the Government, through the definition of social, health and economic policy, which determines the roles that nurses will play
- our employers, who employ us to perform certain roles
- service users, who have first-hand experience of nursing and midwifery and have expectations of the way nurses act and carry out their duties
- the general public and the media, who construct certain images of nurses and midwives as expedient
- others in the profession, who set the culture of nursing as it is practised
- other professions, who have their own views of the role and function of a nurse.

Pre-registration professional education is designed to enable the novice recruit to gain the attributes of a professional. Along the way they are socialised by exposure to the values and ethics of practice and to practice itself so that they adopt the behaviour and practices that make them 'look' like a nurse. This process continues after registration, where the new practitioner is continually absorbed into the system of nursing where they work, in order that the system is perpetuated.

Fundamentally, professional practitioners belong to a 'profession', an occupation that is characterised by:

- requiring higher education
- having a body of knowledge and theory
- providing vital human and social services
- possessing autonomy, control and accountability
- involving altruistic life work
- having a code of ethics. (Hoffart and Woods 1996).

Nursing can be seen to have elements of all of these characteristics, and therefore claims to be a profession. But what do these mean in reality?

Activity

Consider each one of these characteristics in terms of:

Your own understanding
A professional practitioner you admire
A professional practitioner you do not admire
Your own practice

Requiring higher education

All professional nursing preparation is now located within the higher education sector, and involves academic preparation to at least diploma level as well as practice learning in clinical settings. Continuing professional development usually enables the practitioner to advance to a Bachelor's degree (if not gained during pre-registration education) or Master's degree, with many nurses now gaining doctoral level qualifications via a variety of routes, such as clinical or professional doctorates, in addition to the traditional research route of a PhD or Dphil. Career progression is often, and increasingly, linked to educational achievements, with specialist nurses and nurse practitioners having additional preparation at first degree level, and consultant nurses at Master's level.

Having a body of knowledge and theory

Clearly, no one can claim to be a professional without a body of knowledge sufficient for them to pass through a gateway to registration established by the professional body. The NMC sets standards for educational preparation which all students must achieve if they are to be considered as fit for practice. This also includes a 'declaration of good character' required in addition to having passed assessment in theory and practice. The practitioner is expected to build upon this knowledge base, as continuing professional development is a requirement of continuing registration as a practitioner with the NMC, and is therefore integral to a practitioner's practice. This is encompassed in the notion of lifelong learning as being essential for competent practice. Although the individual can claim to have a knowledge base, there is much debate within the literature as to whether nursing itself has a unique base of 'nursing knowledge' that can be attributed to it. The past three decades have seen the growth in nursing research and the creation of nursing knowledge, drawing on, utilising and interpreting other subjects such as biology, pharmacology, psychology and sociology. In addition, nursing utilises medical knowledge, in itself a 'recombinant' knowledge base of fundamental sciences. However, what is evolving from nursing research, and from nurses' experiential knowledge, is a knowledge base about and for nursing, which explicates the ways in which nurses provide nursing care and influence patient outcomes.

Providing vital human and social services

Nursing care has always been a fundamental human activity, with all societies having people who care for the sick and dying. Professional nursing activity is defined in law, and the first registration of nurses came with the Nurses' Registration Acts of 1919. No one is now allowed to call themselves a nurse without a professional qualification that is registered with the NMC. Moreover, registrants have to re-register triennially, providing notification of their 'intention to practise'. This means that the nursing and midwifery register is a 'live' register of active practitioners.

Possessing autonomy, control and accountability

The NMC has delegated power from the Government to both set the standards of practice and discipline its members. The profession therefore has autonomy over its members, as do the medical and legal professions. Nurses have to demonstrate that they work within acceptable standards of practice, and can be removed from the register if they fail to do so.

Involving altruistic life work

Nursing is seen as a 'vocation' which involves giving of oneself and dedication to a professional ethos of caring for others. Nursing is not seen as a self-serving occupation, but as one that exists for the service of other people. Indeed, the *Code of Professional Conduct* (NMC 2004a) expects the practitioner to 'uphold and enhance the good reputation of the profession'. In many ways, once qualified, the nurse is never off duty, as they are expected to render assistance, within the boundaries of their knowledge and skills, to anyone that requires it, for instance in the event of a road traffic accident, major incident or civil unrest. You are also expected to devote some of your time outside the workplace to ensure that you maintain your competence; this may be in formal educational activities, reading professional journals, or attending conferences.

Having a code of ethics

The nursing profession has had a code of professional conduct since 1992. The latest version (NMC 2004a) updates the previous version and is discussed in more detail below. The *Code of Professional Conduct* lies at the heart of professional practice, and needs to be the main guide within which a nurse or midwife frames their practice.

Professional practice includes the overt and observable characteristics of how a person 'embodies' their profession in relation to the characteristics above. Professional practice is what 'professionals' do within the boundaries imposed by both society and the profession itself. There is an assumption that the individual practitioner accepts these parameters, and in accepting professional status accepts the rights and responsibilities that go with it. The characteristics expected of a registered nurse are encapsulated in the *Code of Professional Conduct: Standards for Conduct, Performance and Ethics* (NMC 2004a).

Summary

- An understanding of the term 'professional practice' comes from many sources including the professional body, the law, its practitioners and society.
- Nursing can lay claim to being a profession because it has preparation though higher education, a definable knowledge base, autonomy, registration, altruism, public service and a code of ethics.
- Nurses are expected to practise to standards laid down by the Nursing and Midwifery Council.

The Nursing and Midwifery Council *Code of Professional Conduct: Standards for Conduct, Performance and Ethics* (2004)

The Nursing and Midwifery Council, within its mission of 'protecting the public through professional standards', is charged with regulating the standards of practice of nurses, midwives and specialist community public health nurses. The Council publish the *Code of Professional Code: Standards for Conduct, Performance and Ethics* (2004a) as a way of ensuring that all registrants are aware of the standards they are expected to uphold within their practice. The Council also has the power to investigate contravention of the code of professional practice and to discipline misconduct through its Fitness for Practice panel. This includes suspension or removal from the register, and therefore has serious implications for a practitioner's working life.

Activity

When did you last read the *Code of Professional Conduct*?
How does the *Code of Professional Conduct* influence your practice?
From memory, how much of it can you remember?

The purpose of *The NMC Code of Professional Conduct: Standards for Conduct, Performance and Ethics* (2004a) is to:

- inform the professions of the standard of professional conduct required of them in the exercise of their professional accountability and practice
- inform the public, other professions and employers of the standard of professional conduct that they can expect of a registered practitioner.

Within this framework, the NMC says:

- As a registered nurse, midwife or specialist community public health nurse, you must:
  — protect and support the health of individual patients and clients
  — protect and support the health of the wider community
  — act in such a way that justifies the trust and confidence the public have in you
  — uphold and enhance the good reputation of the professions.
- You are personally accountable for your practice. This means that you are answerable for your actions and omissions, regardless of advice or directions from another professional.
- You have a duty of care to your patients and clients, who are entitled to receive safe and competent care.
- You must adhere to the laws of the country in which you are working.

Box 8.1 shows the NMC (2004a) *Code of Professional Conduct: Standards for Conduct, Performance and Ethics.*

Box 8.1   Nursing and Midwifery Council *Code of Professional Conduct: Standards, Performance and Ethics.*

As a professional nurse or midwife, you are personally accountable for your practice. In caring for patients and clients, you must:

- respect the patient or client as an individual
- obtain consent before you give any treatment or care
- protect confidential information
- cooperate with others in the team
- maintain your professional knowledge and competence
- be trustworthy
- act to identify and minimise risk to patients and clients.

In addition, the NMC recommends that a practitioner has professional indemnity insurance.

Previously published in NMC (2004a) *Code of Professional Conduct.* Available at www.nmc-uk.org

Activity

Take some time to think about each of the seven statements within the *Code of Professional Conduct* and how you, as a nurse, undertake these in your practice.

I will consider each of these clauses in turn and draw your attention to the main issues relating to each one. However, it is beyond the scope of this book to debate these issues in full. References are given throughout to extra sources of information, and a list of appropriate further reading is provided at the end of the chapter. First though, I need to consider the feature of the *Code of Professional Conduct* that relates to all of its individual clauses, that of accountability.

Accountability

The overarching feature of professional practice is the personal accountability of the practitioner. Being accountable basically means to be responsible for something or someone (NMC 2004a p. 13), and further says 'you are answerable for your actions and omissions, regardless of advice or directions from another professional' (NMC 2004a p. 4). This puts clear responsibility on the individual practitioner for the actions they take in giving care to other people, and requires them at all times to be able to justify their decision-making.

Nurses' accountability is also set within the framework of clinical governance, which, according to Tilley and Watson (2004 p. xiv) 'brought accountability to clearer focus and, on the other hand, changed the nature of accountability'.

Caulfield (2005) identifies four 'pillars' that make up a framework of professional accountability, deriving from different types of authority in nursing practice:

- professional
- ethical
- law
- employment.

Professional accountability

Caulfield (2005) suggests that professional accountability derives from being part of a profession and is framed within the standards and guidelines for practice issued by the Nursing and Midwifery Council. Professional accountability therefore provides a framework for professional practice within which the nurse sets their own practice.

Ethical accountability

Codes of ethics arise from within the society we live in and derive from the moral basis on which we live our lives. Ethical values also come from the individual practitioner, and result from aspects such as religion, education and the values we grow up with in our families and local communities. Hence, although there are ethical values that can be said to be common, such as a prohibition on killing or torturing, each person then relates these to their own experiences to form their own ethical code and moral values base.

This is significant in nursing because the nurse–patient relationship is one of trust, where the patient needs to believe that a nurse is acting in their best interests and will not do them any deliberate, or even unconscious, harm. The cases of Beverley Allitt, a nurse, and Harold Shipman, a general practitioner, are probably the most famous instances in recent times of professionals overstepping ethical codes of practice in deliberately using incorrect doses of drugs to kill their patients. This suggests that their personal codes of ethics were out of keeping with those normally accepted by society, and led them to believe they could take decisions on behalf of their patients which were actually outside their responsibility.

Health care practitioners are allowed to have conscientious objections to taking part in some forms of therapy and may refuse, on these grounds, to look after some patients, for instance those women undergoing a termination of pregnancy. Caulfield (2005 p. 6) suggests that it is important for all nurses to have a clear understanding of their own values as, she says, this will 'enable the nurse to recognise where these are challenged by different values held by others in nursing practice'. This is important in terms of being able to stand up for high standards of care, or challenging others who might not have the same value base, such as those who discriminate against other people or who are negligent in their practice, or even do harm to others deliberately. This may involve the nurse needing to draw poor practice, or standards to other people's attention, or even lead to the need for 'whistle-blowing'.

Law

The two systems of law in the United Kingdom (civil law and criminal law) provide a framework of rules, regulations and cases that determine how we behave in society. Civil law sets out the arrangements that apply between private parties, whereas criminal law deals with the rules established by Acts of Parliament. Civil law would apply, in nursing, in areas of negligence or lack of consent, for example, or when a nurse is injured at work and the nurse sues her employer. In these cases, compensation in monetary form can be imposed by the judge hearing the case. Cases in criminal law may relate, for example, to issues such as access to treatment, detainment under the Mental Health Acts or decisions about health care where a person is not deemed competent to make their own decisions. Penalties under criminal law can be fines, community service or imprisonment.

Nurses are not allowed to break the law in the course of their practice, but if they do they may be subject to legal proceedings. Many nurses and midwives also find themselves being part of legal proceedings when patients they have cared for take action against their employers, such as in medical negligence cases. Other practitioners may be part of proceedings against patients or clients, such as in cases of child protection, where they are asked to testify for public authorities against carers or other members of a family.

Legal accountability for nurses therefore has implications for the standards of record-keeping of every practitioner, as these will provide evidence of the actions and decisions made by them. Standards of record-keeping will be considered later in this chapter.

Employers

A contract of employment sets out the relationship between the nurse and his/her employer in terms of the responsibilities and rights of each party. The expectation of the employer may be couched in the job description written for the person's role, procedures and protocols relating to specific activities and the disciplinary procedures established within the organisation. Employers also have expectations of standards of professional behaviour and the ways in which professionals conduct themselves at work.

Equally, the employee has expectations and legal rights under employment law relating to the conditions at work, health and safety, hours of work and what they are asked to do within their role. The contract of employment is a legal contract, and therefore can be enforced in law, on both sides.

Summary

- Accountability is seen as a key feature of professional practice.
- Caulfield (2005) identifies four pillars of accountability:
  - professional accountability deriving from the Nursing and Midwifery Council
  - ethical accountability deriving from the rules of society
  - legal accountability deriving from civil and criminal law
  - employer liability deriving from the relationship between the employer and employee.

Activity

Consider the elements of your professional role against the four pillars of accountability.

Is there any action you need to take to ensure that you are practising effectively as a professional practitioner?

The clauses of the *Code of Professional Conduct*

Clause one: respect for the patient and client as an individual

The NMC considers patients, clients and their carers as partners in their care and expects nurses to involve them in any decisions being made. This is part of the wider Governmental agenda of service user participation, in attempting to ensure that health and social care services are responsive to the needs of the population. Nurses can achieve this by identifying, with the patient, their preferences for care and respecting these within professional and legal limits, resources and the goals of the therapeutic relationship. This is expected to be undertaken within 'appropriate professional boundaries' in terms of the relationships with patients and clients, in that all aspects of the relationship must focus exclusively on their needs.

Nurses are expected to take a value-free approach to their patients in promoting and protecting their interests and dignity at all times, irrespective of:

- gender
- age
- race
- ability
- sexuality
- economic status
- lifestyle
- culture
- religious or political belief.

This includes facilitating access to health and social care, information and support. This means that you must not discriminate between people in the care that you give and nurses are expected to offer care to anyone who needs it. You can report a conscientious objection to your manager if you feel unable to care for a certain individual or client group. However, you must continue to offer care until arrangements are made to relieve you of your obligation and you must continue to practise within the code of professional conduct until that time.

Summary

- Nurses are expected to respect the patient and client as an individual by considering their needs.
- Nurses are expected to maintain appropriate professional boundaries within their relationships with patients and clients.
- Nurses must not discriminate against patients and clients on the grounds of personal beliefs, attributes and lifestyle.

- Nurses can raise a personal conscientious objection to caring for individuals or groups, but must continue to care for them until relieved by another nurse.

Clause two: informed consent

Nurses must obtain consent before giving any treatment.

Activity

What do you understand 'informed consent' to mean?
Who is responsible for obtaining informed consent?
Who can give informed consent?
What sources of advice and information are available to you about informed consent?

Patients and clients have a right to accurate and truthful information about their condition and treatment options, presented in a way that they can understand. Wright and Hill (2003 p. 139) suggest that this information should include:

- the purpose of the investigation or treatment
- explanations of the diagnosis
- options for treatment, including the option not to treat
- the potential benefits and chances of success for different options
- the risks and side-effects of different options
- a reminder that the patient can change their mind at any time
- truthful answers to patients' questions.

This ensures that it is 'informed' consent for treatment that is obtained, as opposed to just consent from the patient to go ahead.

The issue of obtaining informed consent for any patient treatment was clarified in 2001 with the publication of the *Reference Guide to Consent for Examination or Treatment* (DH, 2001a) as part of the strategies outlined in the Government White Paper *Good Practice in Consent: Achieving the NHS Plan Commitment to Patient-centred Consent Practice* (Department of Health 2001b). This is summarised in Box 8.2 outlining the 12 key points of good practice expected by all practitioners.

Informed consent is at the heart of any action that one person does for or with any other person. Prior to clarification in the 2001 legislation, the rules surrounding consent were very fuzzy, with consent for many aspects of treatment being implied simply because a person either turned up for an appointment, took a prescription from a doctor, or said 'yes'. The public outcry and inquiries into the use of post-mortem material retained in Liverpool and procedural irregularities

---

Box 8.2 Twelve key points on consent: the law in England.

(1) Before you examine, treat or care for competent adult patients you must obtain their consent.

(2) Adults are always assumed to be competent unless demonstrated otherwise.

(3) Patients may be competent to make some health care decisions, even if they are not competent to make others.

(4) Giving and obtaining consent is usually a process, not a one-off event.

(5) Before examining, treating or caring for a child, you must also seek consent. Young people aged 16 and 17 are presumed to have the competence to give consent for themselves. Younger children who understand fully what is involved in the proposed procedure can also give consent (although their parents will ideally be involved). In other cases, someone with parental responsibility must give consent on the child's behalf, unless they cannot be reached in an emergency. If a competent child consents to treatment, a parent cannot override that consent. Legally, a parent can consent if a competent child refuses, but it is likely that taking such a serious step will be rare.

(6) It is always best for the person actually treating the patient to seek the patient's consent.

(7) Patients need sufficient information before they can decide whether to give their consent, for example information about the benefits and risks of proposed treatment, and alternative treatments.

(8) Consent must be given voluntarily: not under any form of duress or undue influence from health professionals, family or friends.

(9) Consent can be written, oral or non-verbal.

(10) Competent adults are entitled to refuse treatment, even where it would clearly benefit their health. The only exception to this rule is where the treatment is for a mental disorder and the patient is detained under the Mental Health Act 1983. A competent pregnant woman may refuse any treatment, even if this would be detrimental to the fetus.

(11) No one can give consent on behalf of an incompetent adult. However, you may still treat such a patient if the treatment would be in their best interests.

(12) If an incompetent patient has clearly indicated in the past, whilst competent, that they would refuse treatment in certain circumstances (an 'advance refusal'), and those circumstances arise, you must abide by that refusal.

Source: www.dh.gov.uk/consent

during surgery on babies with heart conditions in Bristol prompted a reconsideration of the rules governing informed consent. This resulted in published guidance for professionals in terms of obtaining consent and the production of a series of guides for different patient groups: adults, children and young people, people with learning difficulties, parents, and relatives and carers, listed in Box 8.3 (available in downloadable format from www.dh.gov.uk/consent). The Government wanted to ensure that consent policies were patient-focused and embedded in the rights of individual patients and their relatives.

The Department of Health provides a model consent policy, together with model consent forms for different groups of patients, which health care providers are expected to adopt. They also publish advice concerning consent for the removal, retention and use of human organs and tissue from post-mortem examinations.

Patients must be legally competent to give consent, give it voluntarily and be informed about what they are consenting to. Patients have the autonomy to refuse treatment on the basis of information given to them, or any other reason that informs their decision. The guidelines make it clear that it is the responsibility of the person giving the treatment to obtain informed consent before the treatment is embarked upon. So for absolute safety, a nurse should get a patient's consent for any treatment that they undertake, not rely on that given to another member of the health care team. However, consent given to another member of the health care team is legally acceptable. Consent can be given non-verbally, orally or in writing. This must also be recorded in the patient's notes.

Where patients are not competent, for example they may be unconscious, or under the influence of mind altering substances, attempts must be made to find out whether decisions about their care were made when they were competent. If this is not apparent, is unavailable or

---

Box 8.3 Government information on informed consent.

Title	Date
Reference Guide to Consent for Examination or Treatment	March 2001
Twelve Key Points on Consent: the Law in England	March 2001
Consent: What You Have the Right to Expect	July 2001
Seeking Consent: Working with Children	November 2001
Seeking Consent: Working with Older People	November 2001
Seeking Consent: Working with People with Learning Disabilities	November 2001
Good Practice in Consent Implementation Guide	November 2001

All available at www.dh.gov.uk/consent

inapplicable, then decisions relating to care must be made in the patient's best interests. This includes emergency situations. Special rules apply to people held under the Mental Health Acts, in relation to children and other vulnerable groups. Nurses caring for people in these groups need to ensure that they understand the issues relating to informed consent, available in the Government booklets and accessed via the relevant websites.

Summary

- Approved practices concerning informed consent procedures are outlined by the Department of Health.
- Informed consent must be obtained before any treatment or investigation is carried out.
- It is the responsibility of the practitioner giving the treatment to obtain consent.
- Consent must be documented in the patient's records.

Activity

Do the informed consent forms used by your organisation comply with those advised by the Department of Health?

Do you need to review your own practice regarding informed consent?

If you work with any of the vulnerable groups mentioned, are you aware of the issues of consent relating to their treatment?

Clause three: confidentiality

Professional confidentiality between patients and the members of the inter-professional health care team is expected as a basic standard of practice. It is often taken for granted by patients that information they give nurses will not be told to others. However, the parameters of professional confidentiality are very complex, and patients do need to be informed about situations when information they provide might be shared with others when it is pertinent to the care they receive.

The NMC (2004a p. 8) says: 'You must treat information about patients and clients as confidential and use it only for the purposes for which it was given.' Not only must you treat information about others confidentially, you also have a duty to protect information from improper use or disclosure: this suggests that you have responsibilities for other members of staff in terms of the ways in which they also share information.

If you need to share information outside the team, for instance to social workers, independent carers, members of the clergy, you must seek permission from the person concerned. The use of information for research purposes also falls under this umbrella.

Threats to and breaches of confidentiality are often unwitting, and because of circumstances and accepted practices as opposed to a deliberate passing on of information.

Activity

What potential opportunities are available for breaches to confidentiality within your own practice?
What steps could you take to avoid these?

Some of these might arise from:

- patient information, assessment and conversations taking place at the bedside; false security comes from drawing the curtains around a bed space
- nursing/patient handovers being given in public, such as at a nursing station or at the end of a bed
- conversations on corridors, stairwells or lifts or within earshot of anyone else
- information disclosed in telephone calls where someone other than the member of the team or intended person is spoken to; this may be a secretary or practice receptionist for instance, or a relative of the patient concerned
- conversations with colleagues in lunch or tea breaks, on public transport or even outside work
- transporting patient records in cars
- written or dictated notes being typed up by someone else
- sending patient records by email
- the siting of computer screens in public areas.

All of these examples can occur as normal practice, yet present opportunities for patient information to go beyond those who have a need to know it. Fundamental to confidentiality are the record-keeping practices of health care professionals.

Summary

- An assumption of confidentiality between patients and practitioners is at the foundation of professional practice.
- Patients may have different understandings of professional confidentiality to that of practitioners.
- Patient information should only be shared with members of the inter-professional team who have a need to know it, and as it relates to the patient's care.
- Many threats to and breaches of confidentiality arise unwittingly.

Record keeping

'The Nursing and Midwifery Council (NMC) believes that record-keeping is a fundamental part of nursing, midwifery and specialist community public health nursing practice.' (NMC 2005 p. 5)

This sentence opens the NMC guidance offered to practitioners on record-keeping practice. The booklet aims to inform practitioners of what is considered to be good practice, as opposed to providing rigid guidelines. The NMC suggests that good record-keeping is a reflection of the standard of professional practice and that it helps to protect the welfare of the patients and clients by promoting:

- high standards of clinical care
- continuity of care
- better communication and dissemination of information between members of the inter-professional health care team
- an accurate account of treatment and care planning and delivery
- the ability to detect problems, such as changes in the patient's or client's condition, at an early stage.

Activity

Consider the way you keep your records at present.

What is good about your record-keeping?
What could be improved?
Do you think that your records fulfil the requirements listed above?

What is a record?

All documents relating to the care of patients and clients will be considered as records and may be required as evidence in a legal matter or complaint. This includes care plans, diaries and birth plans.

Summary

- Good record-keeping is considered to be part of good professional practice.
- A record is any document made relating to a patient or client's care.

Content and style

The NMC provides specific advice on the content and style of practitioners' record-keeping, and draws attention to some legal aspects that are pertinent for good practice. This is shown in Box 8.4.

These guidelines are specific in terms of the quality of records and record-keeping. They draw attention to the nature of records, pointing out that they should only contain *factual* data, not subjective or specu-

---

Box 8.4 Nursing and Midwifery Council guidance on content and style of record-keeping.

Patient and client records should:

- be factual, consistent and accurate
- be written as soon as possible after an event has occurred, providing current information on the care and condition of the patient or client
- be written clearly and in such a manner that the text cannot be erased
- be written in such a manner that any alterations or additions are dated, timed and signed in such a way that the original can still be read clearly
- be accurately dated, timed and signed, with the signature printed alongside the first entry
- not include abbreviations, jargon, meaningless phrases, irrelevant speculation and subjective statements
- be readable on any photocopies.

In addition, records should:

- be written, wherever possible, with the involvement of the patient, client or their carer
- be written in terms that the patient or client can understand
- be consecutive
- identify problems that have arisen and the action taken to rectify them
- provide clear evidence of the care planned, the decisions made, the care delivered and the information shared.

Source: NMC (2005) *Guidelines for Records and Record-keeping.* Available from www.nmc-uk.org

lative data. This does not mean that records must not contain your judgements or impressions, just that these should be based on objective evidence if they are included. They must also be clear to other people, and not contain terms that are not generally understandable, quite a difficult task for a profession that has traditionally abbreviated and used common professional phrases. It is seen as good practice to involve the patient in writing their records, or certainly to share the record with them and ask them about its accuracy. This may avoid problems later as well as ensuring that events significant to the patient are logged, in addition to what you consider to be important. Remember that patients and their relatives may be able to gain access to their records and therefore challenge anything you have written.

Records should be *contemporaneous*, written as you go along, or as soon after care delivery as possible. It is not good practice to save all your record writing to the end of a shift of duty and then try to remember the whole day's care for each patient. They should also be consecutive, and any errors or changes clearly identifiable.

Finally, the NMC gives guidance on the accountability of the recorded entry in terms of it being legible, dated, timed and signed, with the name of the signatory printed at its first occurrence. This enables the care episode and the record to be tracked back to you at a later date – this might be as long as 21 years. It is therefore in your own interest to provide as full and detailed a record as possible, because you may find yourself involved in a complaint, or criminal proceedings at a later date, and need to defend your practice. Records can also be used in professional misconduct cases held in front of the NMC's Fitness for Practice panels.

Activity

Take each one of the points in Box 8.4 and compare your records to these. Ask yourself:

- Is it apparent that I do this?
- What more do I need to do to ensure I am following these guidelines?
- Is there anything I need to do with my colleagues to ensure our records comply with the guidelines?

The above activity can be seen as part of an *auditing* process, which the NMC recommends as routine practice within organisations. They suggest that standards are set internally for record-keeping, and that periodic audit is made against these standards.

Summary

NMC guidelines about the content and style of records relate to:

- their factual content
- the accountability of the professional writing them
- their contemporaneous nature
- their consistency
- their legibility and clarity for anyone reading them.

Legal issues relating to record-keeping

The NMC (2005 p. 9) states that: 'as a registered nurse, midwife or specialist community public health nurse, you have both a professional and legal duty of care'. As a result, they recommend your record-keeping should be able to demonstrate:

- a full account of your assessment and the care you have planned and provided
- relevant information about the condition of the patient or client at

any given time and the measures you have taken to respond to their needs

- evidence that you have understood and honoured your duty of care, that you have taken all reasonable steps to care for the patient or client and that any actions or omissions on your part have not compromised their safety in any way
- a record of any arrangements you have made for the continuing care of a patient or client.

The frequency of entries will be determined by:

- your professional judgement
- local standards and protocols
- the complexity of the patient's case
- deviations from the norm
- increased intensity of care requirements
- patients who are confused or disoriented or generally give cause for concern.

A key point to remember is that courts of law tend to adopt the view that if something is not recorded then it has not been done.

As anyone who has ever had to give evidence in court will agree, it can be a daunting and frightening experience. You are questioned solely on the admissible evidence, and therefore it is definitely in your own interests to ensure that your records provide a true account of the care provided in a case. When cases do go to court, it is often because of an adverse incident, and it is likely that more than one member of the inter-professional team will have been involved. All will have written their own records, and any inconsistencies between these will be closely scrutinised. It is also wise to remember that other people will always defend themselves if their careers are threatened, so try to ensure that your practice falls within the law. This is particularly important if you are taking orders over the phone, or verbally from other health care professionals.

Health care records need to be kept for a minimum of eight years, or, in the case of a child, until their twenty-first birthday. There are also likely to be local protocols established by your employer that you need to be aware of.

As an accountable practitioner you are professionally responsible for any duties delegated to members of the health care team who are not themselves registered. This includes student practitioners and health care assistants. You are responsible for checking the standards of their work, for checking any records they may write and for countersigning these. You are advised against using only your initials in signing records.

Activity

Reconsider your record-keeping practice.

Are there any changes you intend to make now, having read the section on legal issues above?

Summary

- Your records are admissible as evidence in a court of law.
- They should provide clear and accurate records of your care of a patient or client.
- Do not depend on others to defend your practice, especially if you have broken the law.
- Health care records must be kept for a minimum of eight years, or until a child's twenty-first birthday.
- You are accountable for the actions and records written by unregistered health care personnel.

Access and ownership

The advent of the computer age and the Internet has brought with it the need to safeguard how information about individuals is processed and kept, who has access to it, and who can pass it on to others. This is enshrined in law, and expands the notion of confidentiality implicit within the NMC's *Code of Professional Conduct*.

The Data Protection Act 1998

Access to health records is regulated by the Data Protection Act 1998 and gives patients and clients access to both paper-based and com-

---

Box 8.5 The eight principles of good practice in the Data Protection Act 1998.

Anyone processing personal information must comply with eight enforceable principles of good information handling practice. These say that data must be:

(1) fairly and lawfully processed
(2) processed for limited purposes
(3) adequate, relevant and not excessive
(4) accurate and up to date
(5) not kept longer than necessary
(6) processed in accordance with the individual's rights
(7) secure
(8) not transferred to countries outside the European Economic area unless that country has adequate protection for the individual.

Source: Data Protection Act fact sheet. Available at www.informationcommissioner.gov.uk

puter-held records. The DPA gives rights to individuals about infor-mation held on them, and places obligations on those who process that information. The DPA establishes eight principles of good practice, shown in Box 8.5.

Activity

Consider the eight principles of good practice in relation to your own profes-sional practice.

Do you comply with these eight principles?
Are there any areas of your practice you need to change in relation to these?
Are there any wider areas that you need to address at your place of work?

Nurses are most likely to be dealing with personal information about people in their care and their relatives, and therefore have responsibil-ities to ensure that information kept about people is accurate and not shared with those people who are not entitled to have that informa-tion. Moreover, the people that the information is about have certain rights of access to that information and about what happens to it. There are seven rights under the Act, summarised in Box 8.6. Criminal charges may be brought for contraventions against the Act.

Box 8.6   Rights under the Data Protection Act 1998.

There are seven rights under the Data Protection Act:

(1)   the right to subject access
(2)   the right to prevent processing
(3)   the right to prevent processing for direct marketing
(4)   rights in relation to automated decision-making
(5)   the right to compensation
(6)   the right to rectification, blocking, erasure and destruction
(7)   the right to ask the Commissioner to assess whether the Act has been contravened.

Source: www.informationcommissioner.gov.uk

The DPA talks about responsibilities of people 'processing' informa-tion. This relates directly to nurses and anyone else who is delegated with using information collected, whether this is in electronic or paper versions. Furthermore, information must be 'fairly' processed. The DPA identifies six conditions that could be met for personal informa-tion to be considered as being processed fairly; a minimum of one of these must apply. These conditions are shown in Box 8.7.

Box 8.7 The six conditions of fair data processing.

At least one of the following conditions must be met for personal information to be considered fairly processed:

(1) the individual has consented to the processing
(2) processing is necessary for the performance of a contract with the individual
(3) processing is required under a legal obligation (other than one imposed by the contract)
(4) processing is necessary to protect the vital interests of the individual
(5) processing is necessary to carry out public functions, for example administration of justice
(6) processing is necessary in order to pursue the legitimate interests of the data controller or third parties (unless it could unjustifiably prejudice the interests of the individual).

Source: www.informationcommissioner.gov.uk

Activity

Consider the rights and conditions relating to data protection in Boxes 8.6 and 8.7.

What steps do you take within your practice to ensure you are working within the law?
Are there any areas you need to tighten up on?
Are there any areas where you feel there is an issue for your employer that you need to follow up?

Finally, and of extreme importance for nurses, are the provisions made under the Act in relation to any data considered to be sensitive. Data is sensitive if it falls into any one of the following categories:

- racial or ethnic origin
- political opinions
- religious or other beliefs
- trade union membership
- physical or mental health conditions
- sex life
- criminal proceedings or convictions.

Nurses are likely to have access to at least four of these categories as part of the routine data collection made for any patient or client. It is therefore essential that nurses understand the nature of confidentiality in relation to personal information and their own responsibility for the information they have about other people. Sharing this sort of information outside the inter-professional health team may contravene the provisions of the Act and have serious consequences for the person who has done so. The Act therefore imposes extra conditions on the processing of this data, at least one of which must be met:

- having the explicit consent of the individual
- being required by law to process the information for employment purposes
- needing to process the information in order to protect the vital interests of the individual or another person
- dealing with the administration of justice or legal proceedings.

Summary

- Access to personal information is controlled by the Data Protection Act 1998.
- Eight principles of good practice in relation to the nature of data protection are identified within the Act.
- Seven rights are identified under the Act, which provide protection to individuals about whom information is stored. These relate to access; processing; compensation; rectification; blocking; erasure and destruction; and access to the Commissioner.
- Specific provision is made for processing sensitive data; this includes racial or ethnic origin, political opinions, religious or other beliefs, trade union membership, physical or mental health conditions, sex life, criminal proceedings or convictions.

The Freedom of Information Act 2000

The Freedom of Information Act 2000 grants rights of access to anyone to all information not covered by the Data Protection Act 1998; that is, information which does not include patient data.

As a professional practitioner, you may be able to withhold information from a patient or client if you 'believe [it] could cause serious harm to the physical or mental health of the patient or client, or would breach the confidentiality of another patient or client' (NMC 2005 p. 10). You must be able to justify making this decision and record it.

Activity

Can you identify any patients or clients that you have cared for where you feel it would be appropriate to withhold information on the records?

How would you justify and record this decision?

What sort of information do you hold that would be covered by the Freedom of Information Act?

Records are owned by the organisation that employs the person who makes them. This does not mean, however, that anyone who works for the organisation has a right to access them. Professionals must respect the rights of confidentiality of the individual about whom the record is kept, or they may be in contravention of the Data Protection Act 1998. Consent must be gained from the person who is the subject of the record before any information is disclosed, unless the information is being shared with other members of the inter-professional health care team.

The NMC encourages the use of patient-held and parent-held records where appropriate. It also acknowledges that there is sometimes a need for supplementary records to be kept by professional practitioners – for instance, where a specialist community public health nurse is working with a family where there is a child protection concern. Supplementary records must be able to be justified and their existence made clear to other members of the health care team, who should have access to the information contained in them provided it does not compromise patient and client confidentiality.

Records used for research purposes are covered by the same principles of access and confidentiality. Access to records needs to be approved by patients, and usually through protocols for the study submitted to the local research ethics committee.

Computer-held records

The same principles apply to computer-held records as to manual, paper-based records. Safeguards for computer systems need to comply with the Computer Misuse Act 1990. As a professional, you are accountable for ensuring the system you use is secure. This is particularly difficult at a personal level for practitioners working in large organisations where they have neither the knowledge nor the authority to challenge the security of a system in use. However, it is likely to be legally defensible for a practitioner to delegate responsibility for systems' safety to their employer, provided a breach of security does not occur at the point of use. For instance, patients, clients and their relatives should not be able to read a computer screen situated at a ward desk. If you send records by fax or email, you must ensure that they are received by the person they were intended for.

Activity

Have any issues been raised for you in the last section?
How confident are you in the security of computer systems you use?
Could you make any changes to practice that would improve the security?

Summary

- Records not containing personal patient information may be accessed under the provision of the Freedom of Information Act 2000.
- Health care records are owned by the organisation employing the person that compiled them.
- Health care professionals can withhold information if they consider it will harm the patient.
- Patient-held and parent-held records are encouraged.
- Records can be used for research purposes if authorised.
- Computer-held records are subject to the same regulations as all other records.
- Practitioners can be held responsible for breaches of security of computer-held records.

Clause four: cooperation with other members of the inter-professional team

The 'inter-professional team' is seen in a very broad sense, and includes the patient and their carers as well as other professional practitioners and workers from the private and voluntary sectors. Central to this notion of inter-professional cooperation is the recognition of the range of expertise and skills available to provide appropriate packages of care for patients, and that these all contribute to supporting the patient and their family.

Good and effective communication between members, facilitated by shared professional standards and codes of conduct, is key to inter-professional cooperation. All professions are governed by published codes of conduct. Those relating to the allied health professionals (such as occupational therapists, radiographers, operating department practitioners, physiotherapists and dieticians) have been brought into a common framework published by the Health Professions Council (2003). This includes the establishment of protocols for access to health care records as well as verbal conduct and case meetings. Good communication, according to Wright and Hill (2003 p. 133) has been shown to:

- improve patient adherence to treatment
- increase effectiveness of treatment outcomes
- increase patient satisfaction
- increase informed decision-making by patients
- promote respect and empathy between health professional and patient.

It is very easy for communication to be ineffective. Some of the reasons for this might relate to:

- traditional professional boundaries and specialities
- perceived hierarchies between and within the individual professions
- the complexity of the care required
- the differing care environments, such as health service primary and secondary care trusts, private and voluntary residential care, home supported care
- the working patterns of different professions, and their availability, particularly outside 'normal' working hours
- cultural and language problems
- the use of professional jargon
- incomplete record-keeping.

These need to be considered as very real barriers to effective care and strategies need to be established to ensure that their effects are minimised. Wright and Hill (2003) suggest 11 points as foundational for good communication, and these are shown in Box 8.8.

Even when working within a team, a registered nurse remains accountable for their practice under the NMC *Code of Professional*

Box 8.8 Foundations for good communication. Adapted from Wright and Hill (2003 p. 135).

(1) Introduce yourself by name and title. If you are a student, ensure that you tell people this too.
(2) Assess what the patient, or other person, understands and believes.
(3) Avoid jargon, abbreviations and technical words.
(4) Pitch at the appropriate level for the person you are talking to; use short words and sentences wherever possible.
(5) Structure your conversation so that important information is given at the start and end.
(6) Emphasise and repeat important information; summarise any decisions, agreements made or courses of action and check them out with the other person.
(7) Use a structure to communicate information (for example first, second . . .).
(8) Give specific, rather than general health advice when talking to patients.
(9) Maintain eye contact rather than looking at notes, and try active listening. If you make notes as you go along, share these with the other person.
(10) Provide readable leaflets and information for written back-up, but don't assume that the patient will necessarily read them. Always go through the content of the information with them; this is particularly important with drug and treatment information.
(11) Document what you have discussed with the patient, and with other members of the team.

Conduct. This accountability cannot be delegated to others, but certain aspects of care delivery can be delegated to other members of the team. However, you are responsible for ensuring the competence of those to whom you delegate, for the standards and safety of that work, and for providing adequate supervision of the person you delegate to.

Finally, you have a duty to cooperate with any internal or external investigations. These might relate, for instance, to adverse patient incidents, or complaints from patients and their carers.

Activity

How do you communicate with others in the inter-professional team?
What informal methods of communication do you use?
What formal methods do you use?
How effective are they?
Can you think of an example where effective communication made a difference to a patient's care?
Can you think of an example where poor communication resulted in poor care?
Do you need to change anything about the ways in which you communicate with others?

Summary

- Effective inter-professional teamworking is central to good patient care.
- Strategies for communication, including protocols for record-keeping, verbal and other written communication are essential.

Clause five: maintaining professional knowledge and competence

Professional practitioners are responsible for ensuring their knowledge and skills are up to date and their practice is competent, lawful and reflects that knowledge base. As identified in previous chapters, the NMC expects that every nurse, midwife and specialist community public health nurse will regularly take part in learning activities that contribute to their continuing professional development, and to deliver care based on current evidence, best practice and validated research where available. Moreover, nurses are expected to 'acknowledge the limits of [their] professional competence and only undertake practice and accept responsibilities for those activities in which (they) are competent' (NMC 2004a p. 9). If you recognise that you are being asked to do something outside your competence you must obtain help and supervision from a competent practitioner until you and your employer consider that you have acquired the knowledge and skill required.

In 1992 the UKCC published *The Scope of Professional Practice* in which it outlined the conditions under which registered nurses could undertake developing responsibilities beyond the traditional boundaries of practice. It stated that nurses, midwives and heath visitors must ensure that they:

- uphold the interests of patients and clients at all times
- keep their knowledge, skills and competence up to date
- recognise the limits to their own knowledge and skill and take appropriate action to address any deficiencies
- ensure that existing standards of care are not compromised by new developments and responsibilities
- acknowledge their own professional accountability for all actions and omissions
- avoid inappropriate decisions.

At the time, the principles of *Scope* were seen as a revolutionary approach to extending practice boundaries for qualified practitioners that enabled the practitioners themselves to decide what skills and knowledge they needed to support their services for clients. This had previously relied on a system of certificates related to tasks, and often involved nurses who moved jobs in re-doing task competence because the certificates they possessed were not transferable between employing organisations.

In 1997, *Scope in Practice* identified 17 exemplary ways in which *Scope* had facilitated developments throughout the United Kingdom. These demonstrate the impact of locating the responsibility for competence with the practitioners themselves, and illustrate how *Scope* has begun to change the way nurses, midwives and health visitors view their work and to open up a more flexible and professionally challenging way of developing practice.

A follow-up study evaluating the perceptions and impact of *Scope* for professional practice concluded that *Scope* 'provides a set of principles which influence how registered nurses, midwives and health visitors practise. It also provides a framework within which practitioners can:

- justify what they are able to do in order to ensure the effective delivery of care
- identify what they are not in a position to do, due to a lack of skills or knowledge, and how that might be remedied. (UKCC 2000 p. 4)

This exemplifies the ways in which professional nursing and midwifery practice, and professional practitioners, have developed in the past 15 years. There is now an acceptance that nurses and midwives can work within standards established by the professional body, and accept both responsibility and accountability for their practice. This is witnessed in the development of specialist nursing roles, which bring with them additional responsibility and independence for devising and delivering nursing and health care. In addition, we have seen the appointment of nurse consultants, standing alongside medical consultants and those appointed within allied health professions, and independent roles such as nurse practitioners who practise in their own right. These roles would have been unthinkable in the NHS of 20 years ago. They do, however, depend on the two key issues related to maintaining professional competence:

- that practitioners keep abreast of new knowledge and skills in their area of practice and are therefore competent to deliver evidence-based care
- that practitioners acknowledge the limits to their competence.

Activity

How do you know that you are competent to practise?

Central to this creation of independent nursing practice roles was the development of a 'live' register for practitioners established by the UKCC and which led to triennial periodic registration for all practitioners wanting to continue to practise. In order to re-register, practitioners need to attest to their continuing professional development in their notification to practise. The standards for this, set out in the NMC *Post-registration Requirements for Education and Practice* (NMC 2004b), have been discussed and explored in some detail in Chapters 1, 2, 3 and 6. However, it is worth reiterating the *PREP* standards here, as they are fundamental to the demonstration of continuing professional competence. These are:

- **The PREP (practice) standard**; you must have worked in some capacity by virtue of your nursing or midwifery qualification during the previous five years for a minimum of 100 days (750 hours), or have successfully undertaken an approved return to practise course.
- **The PREP (continuing professional development) standard**: you must have undertaken and recorded your continuing professional development (CPD) over the three years prior to the renewal of your registration. All registered nurses and midwives have been required to comply with this standard since April 1995. Since April 2000, registrants need to have declared on their notification to practise form that they have met this requirement when they renew their registration. (NMC 2004b p. 4–5)

You are also responsible for passing your knowledge on to others, such as student practitioners, to help develop their competence.

Clause six: being trustworthy

This relates to both your own personal behaviour, and that which would be expected of anyone who claims membership of a particular profession. The NMC (2004a p. 10) says:

'You must behave in a way that upholds the reputation of the professions. Behaviour that compromises this reputation may call your registration into question even if it is not directly connected to your professional practice.'

To some extent, this means that you are expected to behave in a professional way 24 hours a day. On a more serious note, if you have criminal charges brought against you, have a criminal conviction or are implicated in activities seen as compromising professional standards, you may be investigated through the workings of the Fitness for Practice committee, which is the disciplinary body of the NMC.

Professional behaviour also relates to how you use your registration, for instance you are not allowed to endorse the use of specific products or services. There is a fine line to be drawn here between recommending the use of, for instance, a particular brand of baby milk, and endorsing its use through comparisons with other milks and impressions you may give to your clients. Many drug companies and commercial organisations provide a valuable role in health professional updating and education; this is often accompanied by free lunches or dinners, sample products, visits, trips and conferences. Again, the practitioner needs to consider very carefully whether, in accepting these enhancements, they are in any way compromising their independence, or whether they do in fact maintain the objectivity of the advice they give regarding products. You should always take care to explain the advantages and disadvantages of a range of products, if there is a choice, when giving advice to patients. If you do have an opinion about what might suit the patient best, this should be made on the basis of an assessment of the patient's or client's needs and not on your own preferences or commercial gain.

You must also refuse any gift, favour or hospitality that might be interpreted, now or in the future, as an attempt to obtain preferential consideration. Finally, you must neither ask for nor accept loans from patients, clients or their relatives and friends.

Activity

Can you identify any areas of your practice where you might be in danger, however inadvertently, of falling foul of this clause of the *Code of Professional Conduct*?

What steps can you take to ensure that you do not contravene it?

Clause seven: identifying and minimising risk to patients and clients

The *Code of Professional Conduct* charges the practitioner with the following responsibilities in relation to the environment of care:

- To work with others in the team to promote health care environments that are conducive to safe, therapeutic and ethical practice.
- To act quickly to protect patients and clients from risk where a colleague may not be fit to practise for reasons of conduct, health or competence.
- To report circumstances that could jeopardise standards of practice to a senior person with sufficient authority to manage them, if you cannot remedy the circumstances yourself. This must be supported with a written record.
- When working as a manager you have a duty towards:
  — patients and clients
  — colleagues
  — the wider community
  — the organisation.

When facing professional dilemmas, your first consideration must be towards the interests and safety of patients and clients.

- In an emergency, in or outside the work setting, you have a professional duty to provide care. The care provided would be that reasonably expected from someone with your knowledge, skills and abilities when placed in those particular circumstances.

Indemnity insurance

The NMC recommends that all practitioners who are engaged in advising, treating and caring for patients and clients have professional indemnity insurance. They consider this to be not only in the interests of patients and clients, but also for the practitioner in the event of claims of professional negligence.

Employers may accept vicarious liability for negligent acts and/or omissions by their employees, but this does not extend to activities outside the registrant's employment. Many practitioners have professional insurance as a result of being a member of a trade union or professional organisation such as the Royal College of Nursing. If a practitioner does not have indemnity insurance, the NMC states that: 'a registrant will need to demonstrate that all their clients/patients are fully informed of this fact and the implications this might have in the event of a claim for professional negligence' (NMC 2004a p. 12).

This latter point is particularly important for independent practitioners, such as self-employed midwives or health visitors, who need to arrange separate professional indemnity insurance for their practice.

Guidance for students

The Nursing and Midwifery Council recognises that students cannot be held professionally accountable for their practice, as they are not yet registered as practitioners. However, they provide guidance for students within the NMC *Guide for Students of Nursing and Midwifery* (NMC 2002). It is important to remember that students are expected to be working towards professional practice, and are learning from other practitioners as role models. Therefore, although they are not legally accountable, they are being assessed for their potential as practitioners and must understand their accountability by the end of their programme. Key to your registration is a 'declaration of good character' signed by your programme director. This person will not be able to sign this unless they have the evidence from your assessors, within the university and in practice, that you have developed the characteristics of a professional fit for practice. Contributing to this will be your recognition of the limits of your competence and responsibility, and an awareness of your role as a student.

In relation to your clinical experience, the NMC offers the following guidance:

- Work only within the level of your understanding and competence.
- Always work under the direct supervision of a registered nurse or midwife.
- Although you cannot be held *professionally* accountable by the NMC, you may be held accountable by your university or in law for the consequences of your acts or omissions.
- You must respect the wishes of your patients and clients; they have the right to refuse care from you.
- You must introduce yourself accurately at all times as a pre-registration student and not lead people to believe you are a registered practitioner.
- Do not participate in any procedure for which you have not been fully prepared or supervised, even if it is an emergency.
- If you want to use patient information in a written assignment, do not use any material that could lead to the patient being identified.

You must get permission to use patient records, be under supervision when you do so, and not use any information for a purpose that it was not given for.

- Any written record you make in a patient's notes must be countersigned by a registered practitioner.
- Be aware of the local procedures for dealing with complaints.
- If anyone indicates dissatisfaction with the treatment or care they are receiving you should report it immediately to the person supervising you or another appropriate person.

Summary

- You cannot be held professionally accountable for your actions and omissions as a student by the NMC.
- You can be held responsible for your practice by your university and in law.
- Your programme director needs to sign a 'declaration of good character' to support your registration. This will be based on your conduct in practice and education throughout your programme.
- The NMC offer students guidelines for their practice.

Chapter summary

This chapter has set professional development within the context of professional nursing practice. Completing the activities in this chapter will have provided you with a good analysis of the way you practise within the rules and regulations that bind professional practice. These derive not only from the Nursing and Midwifery Council but also from the wider rules of society, such as ethics and the law, and from the relationships you have with people as patients, and your responsibilities to them. In turn, this analysis will help you to identify any professional development needs that arise from any questions you have, or deficits in your knowledge and skills.

Professional practice is a complicated business, framed within a complex network of expectations. Once we are qualified as a nurse or midwife, we are expected to practise within these expectations; professional education is designed to enable the student practitioner to adopt these professional attributes so that they can be trusted by society to behave appropriately.

One of these expectations is that the practitioner will continue to grow within their role, to acquire new knowledge and develop their own, and others', practice throughout their lifetime, so that the public has the confidence that they are receiving the best, and most up-to-date care possible.

Practising as a professional, therefore, has as part of it, a commitment to professional development. These are inextricably linked, as competence as a practitioner will decline if the individual does not develop. Professional development and an awareness of the changes in practice and contemporary knowledge results from reflection on practice. The reflective practitioner is likely to be a safe and competent practitioner, as they constantly explore and challenge their decisions in practice and the experiences they have as a professional.

References

Caulfield, H. (2005) *Accountability*. Blackwell Publishing, Oxford.

Department of Health (2001a) *Reference Guide to Consent for Examination or Treatment*. Her Majesty's Stationery Office (HMSO), London.

Department of Health (2001b) *Good Practice in Consent: Achieving the NHS Plan Commitment to Patient-centred Consent Practice*. HMSO, London.

Health Professions Council (2003) *Standards of Conduct, Performance and Ethics*. HPC, London.

Hoffart, N. and Woods, C. (1996) Elements of a professional nursing practice model. *Journal of Professional Nursing*, 12, 354–364.

Nursing and Midwifery Council (2002) *Guide for Students of Nursing and Midwifery*. NMC, London.

NMC (2004a) *Code of Professional Conduct: Standards for Conduct, Performance and Ethics*. NMC, London.

NMC (2004b) *The PREP Handbook*. NMC, London.

NMC (2005) *Guidelines for Records and Record-keeping*. NMC, London.

Tilley, S. and Watson, R. (2004) *Accountability in Nursing and Midwifery*. Blackwell Publishing, Oxford.

UKCC (1992) *The Scope of Professional Practice*. UKCC, London.

UKCC (1997) *Scope in Practice*. UKCC, London.

UKCC (2000) *Perceptions of the Scope of Professional Practice*. UKCC, London.

Wright, J. and Hill, P. (2003) *Clinical Governance*. Churchill Livingstone, Edinburgh.

Webliography

www.dh.gov.uk/consent
www.informationcommissioner.gov.uk
www.nmc-uk.org

Index